GRENDEL AND HIS MOTHER
Healing the Traumas of Childhood through Dreams, Imagery and Hypnosis

by
Nicholas E. Brink

Imagery and Human Development Series
Series Editor: Anees A. Sheikh

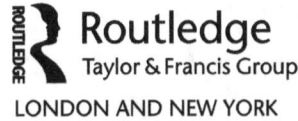

LONDON AND NEW YORK

First published 2002 by Baywood Publishing Company, Inc.

Published 2018 by Routledge
2 Park Square, Milton Park, Abingdon, Oxon OX14 4RN
52 Vanderbilt Avenue, New York, NY 10017

First issued in paperback 2018

Routledge is an imprint of the Taylor & Francis Group, an informa business

Coyright © 2002 Taylor & Francis

All rights reserved. No part of this book may be reprinted or reproduced or utilised in any form or by any electronic, mechanical, or other means, now known or hereafter invented, including photocopying and recording, or in any information storage or retrieval system, without permission in writing from the publishers.

Notice:
Product or corporate names may be trademarks or registered trademarks, and are used only for identification and explanation without intent to infringe.

Library of Congress Catalog Number: 2002018277

Library of Congress Cataloging-in-Publication Data

Brink, Nicholas E., 1939-
   Grendel and his mother : healing the traumas of childhood through dreams, imagery, and hypnosis / by Nicholas E. Brink.
      p. cm. - - (Imagery and human development series)
   Includes bibliographical references and index.
   ISBN 0-89503-262-7 (cloth)
   1. Adult child abuse victims- -Rehabilitation. 2. Dreams- -Therapeutic use. 3. Imagery (Psychology)- -Therapeutic use. 4. Hypnosis--Therapeutic use. 5. Psychic trauma in children. I. Title. II. Imagery and human development series (Unnumbered)

RC569.5.C55 B755 2002
616.85'822390651- -dc21   2002018277

All artwork for *Grendel and His Mother* was done by Benjamin Ruhe.

ISBN 13: 978-0-415-78374-3 (pbk)
ISBN 13: 978-0-89503-262-1 (hbk)

Dedication

To Phillip Rouse who first introduced me to hypnosis, guided imagery, and dreamwork and to Tulsi Saral who gave me permission to write this book.

Table of Contents

Foreword
   L. Michael Bell ix

Preface xvii

Acknowledgments xxiii

Chapter

I   The Imagery of Dreams, Hypnosis, and Myth. 1
           Dreams 1
           Hypnosis 2
           Myth 4

II   The Lineage of Hrothgar: Dissociation from Trauma. 7
           The Nature of Trauma 8
           The First Generation: Exacting Tribute 10
           The Second Generation: Seeking to Please. 13
           The Death of Scyld: The Time for Dissociation 15
           The Third Generation: The Payoff of Success 17
           The Fourth Generation: Becoming Established 20

III   Grendel, Our Despair 23
           Grendel of the Borderlands. 23
           Grendel, The Descendant of Cain 24
           The Grendel of Envy 25
           The Grendel of Self-Blame 27
           God and Abuse 28
           Attacked While Asleep 29
           Grief 30
           Further Attacks 31
           Withdrawal to Outlying Buildings. 32
           The Spirit is Broken 33
           The Treasure-Throne is Safe 34
           Prayers to Heathen Shrines 35

vi / GRENDEL AND HIS MOTHER

IV	The Coming of Beowulf	39
	Beowulf Comes from Across the Sea	39
	Beowulf Comes Unexpectedly	41
	The Sentry Trusts Beowulf	43
	Beowulf's Weapons are Left at the Door	45
	Hrothgar's Chieftain Trusts Beowulf	49
	Hrothgar Knows, Trusts, and Appreciates Beowulf	52
	Beowulf Proclaims His Prowess	56
	Hrothgar Saves Face	59
	Unferth's Jealousy	62
	Wealhtheow Nurtures	66
V	Beowulf's Preparation for Battle	71
	Hrothgar Leaves, Entrusting Heorot to Beowulf	71
	God is Recognized—The Divine Inspiration	75
	Beowulf Lays Down His Weapons	79
	Beowulf's Men Fall Asleep	84
	Only Beowulf Remains Awake	88
VI	The Death of Grendel	93
	Grendel Enters Heorot	93
	Grendel Destroys the Door of Heorot	93
	Grendel Devours a Geat	95
	The Death of Grendel	97
	Beowulf Rises	97
	Beowulf Grips Grendel	99
	Everyone is Seized in Panic	103
	The Hall Stands	105
	The Geats Brandish Their Swords	107
	The Wound	110
VII	The Celebration	113
	Grendel's Arm is Displayed	113
	The People Rejoice	115
	Tracking the Blood of Grendel	117
	A Poet Immortalizes Beowulf	119
	Hrothgar Arrives	121
	The Celebration Gifts	123
	A Ballad is Sung	124
	Wealhtheow Arrives	126
	Flushed with Wine	127
VIII	Grendel's Mother	129
	Grendel's Mother	129
	Grendel's Mother Enters Heorot	131
	Grendel's Mother Seizes Aeschere and Runs	132
	Hrothgar is Broken Hearted	133
	Beowulf Learns of the Night	135

	Beowulf Accepts the Challenge	137
	Following the Blood of Aeschere	139
	Arriving at the Lake	141
	Beowulf's Preparation to Dive	144
IX	The Death of Grendel's Mother	149
	Getting to the Bottom	149
	The She-Beast's Awareness	151
	Grabbed by the She-Beast	152
	The She-Beast's Den	154
	The Beginning of the End	155
	The Warrior and Beast Grapple	157
	Finding the Needed Weapon	160
	Hrothgar Returns Home	162
	Beowulf Gathers the Evidence	163
X	The Final Celebration	167
	Beowulf Swims Ashore	167
	The Return to Heorot and Queen Wealhtheow	169
	The Audience with the King	171
	The King's Oration	172
	Bedding Down for the Night	175
	Beowulf's Preparation for Returning Home	176
	The Gifts from the King	177
	Setting Sail	178
	In Conclusion	179
References		181
Index		183

Foreword

*L. Michael Bell, PhD**

FROM GRENDEL TO "DUNGEONS & DRAGONS": TOLKIEN'S PATH

J. R. R. Tolkien was such a devout Roman Catholic that it is hard to imagine him being sympathetic with psychology. He forbade his students to use the word "creative" on the rather stiff doctrinal reasoning that there is only One Creator. Though he strove to keep his writing from becoming Allegory,[1] he did privately disclose to an American writer (of a Christian, though less doctrinal, bent) that Gandalf the Wizard in *The Lord of the Rings* represents an angel who has taken human form to help earthly mortals. And, to this reader at least, the elf-queen Lady Galadriel echoes just enough of the Virgin Mary to make a Baptist nervous.

Luckily, a powerful imagination can get swept away, even beyond the confines of a devoutly believed dogma. Straying? Trespassing? Perhaps just a brief and unwitting liberation. And Tolkien's imagination was stupendous—to a degree unexampled since Shakespeare. Since late childhood he had been inventing fantasy languages—Elvish, for instance. At some point he realized, as lesser imagineers would not, that a language doesn't exist apart from a distinct people—a society, a nation—to speak it. And a people implies a way of life—a culture. So, in early adolescence, he began to invent (in his peculiarly meticulous way) an Elvish culture. Nourished by his fascination with the literature of the Middle Ages—epics, myths, sagas, romances, legends of King Arthur—his imagination led him from one secret world to another. And, like his creation Bilbo the Hobbit, he returned from this voyage laden with treasure for the whole world's mental imagery—not only stunningly original species like Orcs, Ents, and the hideous but unforgettable Gollum, but concepts of Elves and Dwarves greatly enriched by long roaming through Medieval memory.

*Medievalist & Folklorist in the English Department, University of Colorado.

Far from tinkering with fairytale realms, Tolkien was re-imagining the worlds of the larger-than-life heroes of legend and myth. He truly yearned for England to have a "mythology" like that of even Christian Greeks, who can still look upon Mount Olympus and see a "pagan but noble" (his phrase) symbol of their heritage. Or as modern Christian Norwegians can point to rockfalls caused by Thor's hammer eons ago. The Scandinavian landscape is still speckled with ancient names commemorating pagan gods—as we do, a bit unwittingly, in the names *Tuesday, Wednesday, Thursday,* and *Friday.* Even the Salem-like ferocity of Scandinavian Protestantism, which destroyed runic carvings and their suspected makers, couldn't erase the hundreds of variations on place-names like Odense,[2] Torslunda, Fröslunda, Frötuna (for Odin, Thor, Frey, and Freyja), Thisted, or Ulleråker (Tyr, source of "Tuesday," and the obscure Ullr, god of skiing).

Thanks to Icelandic diligence and a large helping of sheer good fortune, many poems and tales of these gods survived not only Christian hostility but centuries of fire and decay, bookworms and theft. And Rome may have been blissfully unaware that some of its early Northern saints had pagan gods peeping out from their very common traditional names: St. Thorlak, the first Icelandic saint, bore a prefix honoring Thor, as did St. Thorfinn of Norway. And St. Ansgar of Denmark has a ringing Viking name meaning "spear of the [pagan] Gods." Before long, the example of these saints gave such names their imprimatur, and the point became moot.

But in England, Christianity had succeeded in eradicating (or co-opting) nearly every trace of the old belief system. "Of English pre-Christian mythology we know practically nothing," Tolkien observes. "Christmas" replaced the pagan midwinter festival of "Yule"; "Holymonth," hallowing the harvest, was bumped by "November"; age-old tales of heroes like Ingeld were extinguished, and of many others—Sigemund, Waldere, Ongentheow, Hnaef—only scraps remain, often in *Beowulf. Easter* is a rare exception, keeping the name of the pagan goddess of Dawn, Eostre,[3] named for the direction of the returning sun.— Tolkien must have sensed, subconsciously, that sharing a god with a Middle Eastern origin, even if He is one's Only True God, isn't quite as satisfying as a sacred heritage rooted in one's own soil. To borrow his own phrase for Beowulf's author, he wished for England a story of "a past, pagan but noble and fraught with a deep significance." Perhaps the Knights of the Round Table had become too overtly Christian, too religiously specific, to fill the bill. So Tolkien set about constructing his own—a quasi-mythical past, with quasi-sacred dimensions of both time and space, and loosely compatible with his own deep faith.

The poet W. H. Auden—who was about as well-read as a modern poet can be without stuffiness—once observed that Tolkien's invented world went one striking step further: It "satisf[ies]" our sense of historical and social reality." The British are not habitually given to such superlatives as:

No previous writer [emphasis added] has, to my knowledge, created an imaginary world and a feigned history in such detail. By the time the reader has finished the trilogy [and its] appendices . . . , he knows as much about Tolkien's Middle Earth, its landscape, its fauna and flora, its peoples, their languages, their history, their cultural habits, as . . . he knows about the actual world.

Whether they know it or not, few people in today's "actual world" have been untouched by Tolkien's imagination. Even fewer know the extent of its debt to *Beowulf*. The latter point we must briefly postpone for a swift synopsis: Starting in the 1960s with torrential sales of the Ring Trilogy, followed by hordes of imitators, followed by Dungeons and Dragons, and then role-playing movements like the Society for Creative Anachronism; communes and even suburban streets taking names like *Rivendell* and *Lothlorien;* the new (and profitable) fad for Runes; before long, "Star Wars" and then video games—some of whose later spawn would freeze poor Tolkien's blood. A friend who first encountered Tolkien's books in grade school expressed it this way in his late teens:

> The first fantasy role-playing [board] games almost directly copied Tolkien, although not admitting to do so. . . . Elves were the elves of Tolkien,[4] trolls were the trolls, etc. . . . In Dungeons & Dragons, the setting, the races, the culture—was most certainly an almost direct interpretation of Tolkien. In fact, modern D & D has a race called "Halflings" who are, in essence, hobbits. In the first edition, they were even called "Hobbits," and the bestiary included such entries as "Balrog" and "Ent." The Tolkien estate coughed politely, and now they are known [by other names].

The influence of Tolkien's trilogy is hard to overstate. Even beyond its wildly influential brainchildren like those above, it almost singlehandedly revived an extinct category of literature—**so** extinct that early reviewers, trying to describe *LOTR*, fumbled with terms like "sort of a super science-fiction." The category was Fantasy, which within a very short time had dedicated sections in most bookstores. Of all types of writing, it gives freest play to the imagination. And—if this sort of bottom line is required—not too long after it had been raised from the grave by Tolkien and his friend C. S. Lewis (the "Narnia" stories), Fantasy accounted for 10 percent of ALL fiction purchased in the United States for 20 years (1970-1990).[5] After his death, Tolkien was called "the grandfather of the video game industry" by *Publisher's Weekly,* the house organ of the book trade. But, to avoid ending on such a mercenary note, and to cut short this orgy of superlatives (however accurate), *The Lord of the Rings* was recently nominated for the unofficial honor of "Book of the Century.[6] Even ignoring the dozens of foreign translations, it **would** appear that this one man's imagination struck a major chord which resonated with hundreds of millions people.

ENTER GRENDEL

Appropriately but astonishingly, Tolkien's other great achievement—long before writing his trilogy—was to refute the nearly unanimous view that the Anglo-Saxon poem of *Beowulf* was unworthy of being called good literature, let alone great literature. Most scholars had disdained the poem because Grendel, his mother, and the Dragon[7] were the fantasies of a "wild folk-tale," and unworthy of a true epic. ("As if Milton had retold 'Jack and the Beanstalk' in noble verse," Tolkien remarked wryly.) But Tolkien builds his case directly on these monsters. He titled his revolutionary 1936 lecture "*Beowulf:* The Monsters and the Critics"—arguing that the poem derives its very greatness from their symbolic stature: "The universal significance which is given to the fortunes of its hero" is precisely *because* his foes are *in*human[8] enemies of God and mankind as primordial and elemental and lethal as Titans.

Consider the Cyclops, Tolkien proposed. "Of Grendel it is said: *Godes yrre baer* [he bore the anger of God]. But the Cyclops is god-begotten and his maiming is an offence against his begetter, the god Poseidon. [He cites an earlier scholar, Archibald Strong:] "Odysseus is struggling with a monstrous and wicked foe, but he is not exactly thought of as struggling with the powers of darkness. . . . [The Cyclops], by devouring his guests, acts in a way which is hateful to Zeus and the other gods: yet he is . . . god-begotten and under divine protection, and [his maiming] is a wrong which Poseidon is slow to forgive. But the gigantic foes whom Beowulf has to meet are [constantly] identified with the foes of God, . . . the powers of darkness with which Christian men felt themselves to be encompassed.'" In the poem's own words, they are "adversaries of God" [as well as] "enemies of mankind." And Beowulf cleanses his world of them.

A striking fact about Beowulf's first two heroic victories over God's foes is that the Deity all but maintains a hands-off policy. Friederich Klaeber, the authoritative editor of *Beowulf,* has two impressive insights about the second fight: Despite the poem's

> inserted remark that Grendel's mother is less dangerous than Grendel in as much as she is a woman, . . . the second fight is far more difficult for Beowulf than the first, although he is well armed. . . . The she-demon could not be wounded by any weapon except her own. . . . [Yet] God's help consists in nothing else than showing Beowulf the marvelous sword.[9]

And, though the mutual enmity of God and Grendel is reiterated three times in the first battle scene, the deity is absent, even as a "second" or an invisible referee. At the point where one would most expect divine intervention, the central figure decreeing Grendel's destiny is termed "fate" (*wyrd*), a concept quite distinct from God or even the pagan gods.—From this viewpoint, the retroactive credit bestowed on God in the postgame celebrations rings hollow to the alert modern reader, whose keenest impression is of a magnified heroism on Beowulf's part.

In the popular legends of many eras, monsters are conceived of as stupid gluttons, not necessarily hostile. But Grendel, Tolkien emphasizes, "is primarily a . . . physical monster whose main function is hostility to humanity." And the dragon, whom Beowulf sacrifices his own life to slay, personifies "malice, greed, destruction (the evil side of heroic life), and . . . the undiscriminating cruelty of fortune that distinguishes not good or bad (the evil aspect of all life)." "It is just because the main foes in Beowulf are inhuman," he contends, "that the story is larger and more significant than this imaginary poem of a great king's fall."

In his typically reflective way, Tolkien imagines the author of Beowulf, in a time when Christianity was established but pre-Christian cultural memory was still fresh, looking back upon "a past, pagan but noble, and fraught with a deep significance." This poet he visualizes as "an Englishman using afresh ancient and largely traditional material, and using it in an original way." He is worth quoting more fully: In *Beowulf,*

> [T]he use of allusions to old tales, mostly darker and more desperate than the foreground, . . . creates a sense of many-storied antiquity, the illusion of surveying a past, pagan but noble and fraught with a deep significance—a past that itself had depth and reached backward into a dark antiquity of sorrow. [It gives a] sense of perspective, of antiquity with a greater and yet darker antiquity behind. The old dark tales of men and lands beyond the sea echo as from a vast distances.

It diminishes Tolkien's achievement not a bit to say that all of the numerous details in those quotes exactly fit *The Lord of the Rings*—which wasn't even written yet. The tales he "told" the modern world are uncanny in the way they convey a sense of "vast echoing distances," pasts behind pasts beyond pasts, like mountain ranges that grow hazier and dimmer as they recede to the horizon—with even a hint of a vast unseen extending beyond that horizon. And to say that this "ancient and largely traditional material [is] used afresh, and in an original way" is a thundering understatement.

So when we encounter a third comment of his on Beowulf—"[This ancient imagination] has power, as it were, to revive its spirit even in our own times"[10]—and reflect even on the *quantitative* impact of exactly that revival in *LOTR*—what can we say but "amen!"

It is in this deep, spiritually tectonic sense that Tolkien's art was shaped by the art of *Beowulf.* The term "source material" is simply shallow.[11] And this deep spiritual tectonics—a major element of the Tolkien with whom millions resonate—is what Dr. Brink has, for the first time, plumbed and charted in psychotherapeutic terms.

Let's take a more specific sounding:

GRENDEL'S APPROACH TO THE HALL

It's often been observed that a society's mores can be stronger than its formal religion—can alter even a powerful, authoritarian doctrine. In Brazil, Catholics were allowed to eat chicken on Friday because, for so many ages, chicken has belonged so strongly to a different, less meat-like category that mores overrode the Catholic prohibition. In the ancient Germanic society to which Anglo-Saxon culture belonged, even the image of the Christian God and His throne were re-shaped. Hospitality was so (socially) sacred, feasting such a potent symbol, and the chieftain's gift-giving ceremony so deeply important in their mores, that it went without saying. The assumption was too deep for words. And its power to reshape even cosmic concepts was neatly caught in Alvin A. Lee's book title: "Guest-Hall of Eden." Even Paradise was envisioned as a celestial Heorot.

So the statement that Grendel "could not approach the gift-throne" isn't just a throwaway detail. It spotlights him as an outcast. An outcast is hardly a monster; but another, odder detail raises the emotional pitch: The poem devotes 20 lines merely to his approach to the hall. What's the big deal? Was the poet being paid by the word?[12]

It's easy to assume that the spooky old Dark Ages were full of creatures as terrifying as Hollywood's "Alien." Perhaps so. But you will search long and hard for anything in Medieval story whose creepiness endures to this day. As one scholar put it to me: "In the Viking sagas, the hero sees a monster, says, 'Oh, you're a monster.' Bop! No more monster.—But Grendel and his mother, especially that scene when he approaches the hall—it makes me shudder."

The scene has been called "a motif of pure terror"; the sense of Grendel's unearthly menace peaks in this passage. Several times, varied for maximum effect, the poet deploys words like "crept . . . stepped . . . advanced . . . came on . . . ," interlacing them with a shifting collage of images even cinema couldn't capture: Pale night, the sleeping Danes in the darkened hall, Grendel's anger, the "banks of mist," the wakeful Beowulf and his swelling courage, God's curse on Grendel, the wine-hall and its splendid decorations—until the monster reaches Heorot and, in a fury, smashes in the heavy door. He steps onto the "polished floor"—and right then, where a second-rate filmmaker might break the tension explosively, the action stops dead.

Only a consummate tale-spinner could have the confidence in his skill to suspend a climax that way. His spell has been so binding that the next image, an instant before Grendel exultantly scans the hall, has no taint of the comic book or fairy tale: "Out of his eyes came an ugly light, most like to a flame."

The total scene outdoes those of Grendel's mother and the dragon—but not by much. They are the Beowulf poet's deepest art. And what Dr. Brink has plumbed—uniquely—is the even deeper psychological layers of this art, to discover their resonance for modern psychotherapy.

But perhaps these images of "depths" are less fitting than Tolkien's own, in concluding his lecture. It's a bit ironic that they express a feeling for the heart of human psychology with which not even the Vatican would quibble:

> We look down as if from a visionary height upon the house of man in the valley of the world. . . . [The poem] glimpses the cosmic and moves with the thought of all men concerning the fate of human life and efforts.

NOTES

1. Of the artistry in Beowulf he says: "The large symbolism is near the surface, but it does not break through, nor become allegory." [LMB]
2. Birthplace of Hans Christian Andersen. It means "Odin's Shrine." [LMB]
3. By a sad irony, one expurgation did succeed in Iceland. Tuesday, Wednesday, Thursday, and Friday have been bleached into Thirdday, Midweekday, Fifthday, and Fastday. As for poor old Saturn: His day, in modern Icelandic, is Bathday. [LMB]
4. Tolkien restored Elves from the tiny pixies of children's literature to their original nature: Human-size, with extraordinary physical and psychic powers, and who, "though not physically indestructible, do not suffer natural death." (W. H. Auden) [LMB]
5. Lester Del Rey, a Ballantine editor, is credited by the industry with "establishing a new mass market genre" in tones so reverent it suggests a Nobel Prize in Marketing. [LMB]
6. Considering *Esquire* magazine's long tradition of cultural literateness, it's a far from trivial tribute that they named Gollum one of the ten best literary characters of the century—on a short list with, for example, Holden Caulfield of *Catcher in the Rye* and Holly Golightly of *Breakfast at Tiffany's*. [LMB]
7. What is the dragon within? *Loki's Children,* the title of my next book, is about overcoming those monsters within caused by our own foolish actions—monsters we brought on ourselves and for which we need to take responsibility. The monsters, Grendel and his mother, our inner fears and anxieties, are caused by something that acted upon us for which we do not need to take responsibility. The dragon, like Loki's children, we brought upon ourselves. As king, Beowulf needs to protect his people from the dragon enraged by some person or part-within stealing a cup from the dragon guarded treasures. Though the kingly part of us can deny greed, a greedy part of us did steal the cup, and thus we, including the king-with, are responsible. Overcoming those self-created monsters requires death and rebirth of part of ourselves, the death of the inner king, our decision maker, whether the death of the Nordic Pantheon at Ragnarok or the death of King Beowulf and the rebirth of the King, whether as the innocent god Balder or as a new King Wiglaf son of Weohstan. In life we face both kinds of monsters repeatedly and sometimes it is difficult to tell the difference. [NEB]
8. What is the meaning of *inhuman?* I first think of that which is superhuman. The dictionary offers "lacking natural human feeling or sympathy." Another definition or play on words relevant to this book is in-human or that which is within each of us. Grendel and his mother are within us, our fears and anxieties, and the enemies of the God within—the creative, intuitive, inspiring, good and self-actualizing part of us—the

creative in spite of Tolkien's personal beliefs. With the death of Grendel and his mother this God-within is able to flourish. [NEB]

9. This is Klaeber's interpretation, and my interpretation of the variously-translated phrase italicized below. The she-monster has Beowulf pinned to the floor and is about to stab him to death, but "holy God, the Lord all-wise, awarded the mastery; Heaven's Ruler gave right decree *as soon as the hero got to his feet.* He saw amid the war-gear a stately sword. . . ."—God, evidently, helps those who get off their own duffs first. [LMB]

10. This ancient imagination "has power, as it were, to revive its spirit even in our own times." What is this power? It is the fact that this story is alive and relevant within each of us. It constantly affects us, unconsciously evoking deep feelings the same way dreams evoke feelings even when we may not understand them. Hrothgar, Beowulf, Grendel and his mother are alive within us even though we may never have read this ancient poem. Reading the poem resonates with these parts of us. [LMB]

11. In those terms, the only direct borrowing in the whole trilogy is from the medieval French *Song of Roland:* Boromir's last battle and especially his horn. But if Boromir is a Roland-figure, there is no Beowulf-figure, Grendel-figure (even giving Gollum his due), or Grendel's-mother-figure in *LOTR.* (In *The Hobbit,* the ominous but protective figure of Beorn, who shapeshifts from man to bear, can be seen as a Beowulf-figure; "bear" in Anglo-Saxon is *beorn,* and Beowulf's own name stands for "bee-ravager," a typical Anglo-Saxon metaphor for "bear.") Otherwise, the little "source material" which is **not** from Tolkien's own imagination is in details like the stature of elves, or the nature of dragons being to inhabit burial-mounds and lie on piles of gold. [LMB]

12. What is the big deal of twenty line of approaching the hall? We have created these monsters within us by spending many years repressing our early childhood trauma and denying our weaknesses. It often takes years for us to open up to face these inner monsters, a struggle greatly deserving these 20 lines. [NEB]

[LMB] L. Michael Bell
[NEB] Nicholas E. Brink

Preface

The purpose of this book is to increase the reader's understanding of the cause, or one class of causes, of behavioral, emotional, and thought disorders and of the treatment or process of therapy for these disorders with this class of causes.

What is the etiology of behavioral, emotional, and thought disorders? Early research as presented in my beginning psychology courses in college considered and rejected such possible causes as the effect of specific toilet training practices, birth order, and the trauma of divorce. Now, 30 years later, many clients come to me quoting their physician who prescribes medication, saying the cause is chemical changes in the brain. There is some truth to each of these causes, as we shall see.

Let's briefly consider the chemical changes in the brain. The human nervous system is composed of hundreds of billions of neurons. Each neuron sends electrochemical messages or impulses to thousands of other neurons. When an electrochemical impulse reaches the end of an axon of a neuron and jumps across the synapse or gap to the next neuron, this jump is made chemically with chemical neurotransmitters. Much of the neurological and neurochemical research on emotional disorders has focused on the limbic system or the emotional center of the brain. So far, more than 300 different neurotransmitters have been identified. Two of the better-known neurotransmitters are dopamine and serotonin. When you think of all the combinations and permutations of these neurons in combination with the many possible neurotransmitters, the possibilities are astronomical.

When an electrical impulse is repeatedly passed from one neuron to the receptor of the next, the sensitivity of the receptor to the neurotransmitter increases so that it takes less and less stimulation to the receptor for it to "fire" or respond to the neurotransmitter. Within the field of neurology this process of "learning" is referred to as kindling. Kindling "involves progressive increases in electrical (neural) excitability in response to less and less stimulation" (Dubovsky, 1997). With sufficient kindling the response becomes autonomous of the stimulus, i.e., the neuron learns the response so well that it takes no stimulus to trigger it.

The ramifications of the concept of kindling and an autonomous response are many. One logical consequence is that neurology, pharmacology, and psychiatry have searched for chemical means to modify or rekindle the process of neurotransmission at the synapse as a means of decreasing the symptoms of such psychiatric disorders as depression, anxiety, obsessive compulsive disorders, bipolar disorders, and schizophrenia. These sciences have paid little concern to the original stimulus that triggers the neural response. The physician who says the emotion is caused by a chemical change in the brain is ignoring the stimulus that initially triggers the reaction, as well as what is going on in the cognitive parts of the brain. Let's consider a simple example.

Whenever infant Jason spits out food while his father feeds him, his father sighs. Children, even verbal children, respond with feelings before they respond with words. Jason may not understand the meaning of his father's sigh but if he were able to express himself verbally, he might say, "Daddy is upset," "I'm a bad boy," "Daddy doesn't understand I'm full," or "Daddy doesn't understand I don't like the taste." But since Jason is preverbal and does not have the vocabulary to mediate these thoughts, he just feels anxious, scared, or trapped in the situation. He may have already learned from experience that daddy's sigh is going to turn to anger, escalated by Jason's anxiety and refusal to eat and father's frustration. The feeling of anxiety is kindled, i.e., it becomes a learned response to dad's sigh and soon the sighs of others—the stimulus. Each time Jason hears a sigh he becomes anxious. Eventually he may feel anxious even without hearing a sigh. The kindled anxiety then becomes autonomous of the stimulus.

More concerned with the resulting anxiety than the stimulus of a sigh or the meaning of the sigh to Jason, psychiatry's solution is to provide medication to change the chemistry at the synaptic level of the emotional center of the brain to diminish the feeling of anxiety. This solution ignores many aspects of what was learned. Jason may have learned that "people are unhappy with me" or "I can't do anything right." He may lack self-confidence and he may not have the cognitive and verbal ability to put such beliefs into words, but these beliefs can still be unconsciously part of him. In considering the neural process of kindling, therapy to uncover and help Jason change his way of thinking and his self-beliefs seems to be another logical conclusion. Simply prescribing medication ignores such internal language and beliefs that exist in other more cognitive structures of the brain left unaffected by the medication.

Uncovering and changing such internal language is the goal of cognitive behavioral therapy, but uncovering and replacing such ways of thinking are more easily said than done, especially when such self-beliefs are unconscious. The tools of dream work, mental imagery, and hypnosis are most effective in facilitating such uncovery and change. In considering the stimulus that triggers an emotional response, several factors need to be considered. First, the stimulus is the way an event is perceived and interpreted. Jason's father's sigh likely means something different to Jason than it does to his father. Some children may not even notice a sigh. To others it may have some other meaning. In therapy, what is important is what the sigh means to Jason. To Jason the sigh can be considered a trauma, though to Jason's father it was a simple honest and gentle expression of his frustration.

Second, the stimulus that triggers an emotional response needs to be described in Jason's own words, images, or experience. Hypnotic time regression can help an individual identify the stimulus when the experience has been forgotten, repressed, or preverbal. When the learning or kindling of an emotional response was preverbal, the uncovered stimulus may be in the form of an image or other sensory experiences. Considering all of the senses can be of use. When a person is verbal the experience is generally verbal or auditory but experiences are often visual or imaginal in nature. Other times the stimulus may be tactile, olfactory, or even gustatory.

Third, Jason needs to find the right words to describe the emotional response to the stimulus. The hypnotic technique of instructing the client, "Let your adult self go back and be with your younger self and help your younger self find the right words to explain how you feel," is effective in identifying those feelings. Putting such experiences and feelings into words helps an individual gain some control over the experience.

Fourth, the repeated behaviors and attitudes of others that define the stimulus for the emotional response can be considered traumatic to the individual, and since such trauma is external to the individual, the individual does not or should not have to take responsibility for it. Such external stimuli are the class of causes of behavioral, emotional, and thought disorders to be considered by this book and will be referred to as the trauma. As you can imagine, the breadth of possible trauma is enormous, extending from the severe trauma of physical and sexual abuse and abandonment to such simple behaviors as a simple sigh, or such verbal comments as "after all I've done for you" or "where were you when the brains were passed out?"

Another class of causes, those decisions made by the individual to do something or be a certain way, behaviors and beliefs that are determined by the individual and for which the individual needs to take responsibility, will be the subject of a second book, *Loki's Children*.

Fifth, the traumatized individual needs to identify in affirmative terms what he or she needs to determine alternative behaviors and attitudes. I once heard a story from another psychologist: "A child comes into my office, touches something and I say 'no.' What does the child do but to run off to touch something else. Again I say 'no.' In no time at all, the child is racing around the office touching everything looking for a 'yes.'" This story was told to describe the etiology of hyperactivity, but it also is a good example of a problem in the process of learning or kindling, and relearning or rekindling. When we become aware of some dysfunctional or unwanted response to some stimulus or even an autonomous behavior, we may seek to refrain from the response, but we may have no idea what to replace it with. The "yes" can remain a mystery. Uncovering the history of the kindled behavior is important, but finding a healthy or functional alternative for rekindling is at least as important. To help an individual find the "yes," another hypnotic technique has been found to be very effective: "Let your adult self go back and be with your younger self and help your younger self find the right words to describe what you need." Jason might say, "Dad, I need you to be patient" and "Dad, I need you to understand that I don't like the taste, I need you to be more understanding." For Jason to say, "I need dad not to sigh," tells nothing about the alternative of what he does need.

Sixth, in stating what we need from dad, mom, or some other significant figure, we are not talking directly to our father or mother but to our inner father, mother, or other archetype. Talking to this inner part of ourselves helps us to integrate that archetype. As these internal images become better integrated in a healthy manner, we become the healthy father and mother to others in our lives. Becoming aware of these personal changes is an important part of the healing process.

If Jason as an adult is successful in changing the way he thinks or believes, thus "rekindling" the cognitive parts of the brain, and nothing changes in the emotional portions of the brain, he will continue to experience the anxiety response. On the other hand, if medication changes the anxiety response but Jason does not change the way he thinks or believes, when he stops taking the medication the anxiety will return. It takes changing both the thinking and the emotional responses to effect deeper change.

This book offers psychotherapeutic ways through hypnosis, guided imagery, and dream work to uncover our dysfunctional self-beliefs and internal language, and to learn functional and healthy alternatives for rekindling ourselves.

As mentioned above, there are at least two different classes of causes of behavioral, emotional, and thought disorders that for resolution determine different courses of therapy. The purpose of this book as described above addresses the first of these two "causes." My second book, *Loki's Children,* will address the second. Though it may be difficult or impossible to separate these two causes in the therapy room, the distinction does have implications for the course of and the techniques used in therapy.

In *Grendel and His Mother* something has happened external to the individual, outside of his or her control, that has caused the tormenting behavioral, emotional, or thought disorder. The ancient Old English myth of Beowulf offers us a map for our journey through the unconscious mind to overcome this torment, first to give us strength to overcome the more immediate torment of the behavioral, emotional, or thought disorder, our Grendel, and then to uncover and overcome the deeper cause of this torment, Grendel's mother. Why use a myth as a map of this journey? Myths, the dreams of our ancient ancestors, like any dream, describe the process of the unconscious mind. Whereas an individual dream is specific to an individual, a myth of the culture describes the unconscious process on a more universal level applicable to all of us.

Jason, now as an adult, is suffering anxiety and panic attacks; he is dissociated from the cause of these panic attacks just as Hrothgar, the great king in the story of Beowulf, is dissociated from the cause of the emotional pain of his original abandonment. Hrothgar's immediate torment, i.e., Jason's panic attacks, is seen in the form of the monster Grendel who nightly attacks his great hall and kills the King's retainers. The fact that Jason has initiated therapy suggests that his inner warrior has been called upon and is preparing to face and destroy his tormenting anxiety, just as the great warrior Beowulf is summoned to save Hrothgar from Grendel. With this victory Beowulf is able to celebrate his authority over Grendel, just as Jason celebrates his victory over his anxiety, only to have another monster, Grendel's mother, arrive to cause further torment. After tracking Grendel's mother back to her den in the murky waters of a monster infested lake, Jason's unconscious mind, the warrior Beowulf, succeeds in killing this second monster. When Jason uncovers the original, unconscious source of his torment, the sighs of his father, he can truly free himself from this torment. Each line of this ancient poem has something to offer in explaining the course of therapy to overcome that which has tormented us since our early years, that something which is outside of our domain of responsibility and which we have forgotten.

Similarly, the ancient Greek myth of *Twelve Labors of Hercules* also describes a journey of overcoming such torment. As Hercules succeeds in completing twelve superhuman tasks, he is able to overcome the torment caused him by his stepmother, the Goddess Hera, and thus becomes a god in the Greek pantheon.

The second cause of behavioral, emotional, and thought disorders is well illustrated in the ancient Nordic myth of *Loki's Children*. In this second category of problems, rather than the cause arising from outside of ourselves, the problems are caused by the decisions we make in determining who we are and what we do that turns out not to be so wise. The trickster god within us, Loki, begins to torment us and finds ways to make us face the not-so-wise way we have become or the not-so-wise things we do. He torments us with three monsters, the three children of Loki: Jormungand, our fear; Hel, our guilt; and Fenrir, our obsessive worry. As we are forced to face these three monsters within us, we eventually die and are reborn in the new innocent Balder. The process of therapy to overcome our fear, guilt, and obsessive worry caused by our unwise decisions, whether conscious or unconscious, leads us to face the final battle of death, Ragnarok, and rebirth lifting us then to a new level of life.

In a similar Irish myth, the high king Fergus, when confronted by Esirt, the Leprechaun King's poet and our internal trickster, admits that he made a poor decision by being unfaithful to his Queen. Esirt's taunts eventually lead to Fergus's death, while facing a great lake monster, and his rebirth as the even greater and more famous King Fergus. This story is found in the ancient Irish myth of *The Death of Fergus Mac Leide*. Since these behavioral, emotional, or thought disorders are caused by our own unwise decision making, a part of us has to die before we are able to rise to new heights, whereas when we are not required to take ownership of our problem when caused by something outside ourselves, such death is not necessary.

Why do we make such unwise decisions? Sometimes it is because of things that happened to us early in life. "I am not going to be angry like my father was," or "I am not going to let people walk over me like my mother did," are such decisions. Each of us make these decisions for which we need to take responsibility yet these decisions are based on experiences from outside of ourselves and for which we need not take responsibility. Thus, the distinction between these two causes of disorders is lost, yet facing problems with this distinction in mind opens doors in self-understanding and facilitates the journey of personal growth. The intersection between these two etiologies and the flow back and forth in the process of therapy will be considered in *Loki's Children*.

Nicholas E. Brink
Coburn, Pennsylvania
nbrink@imaginalmind.com

Acknowledgments

I first thank the clients of my 30 years of practice who have been my teachers and I their student. My gratitude also goes to Sabrina Kirby who read and edited this book twice and had to deal with my life-long affliction of dyslexia, to my lunchtime friend, Bernie Olszowy, whose good listening skills helped clarify many thoughts, and to my wife, Toni, who put up with my affair with writing.

I also thank the readers of the manuscript who gave me constructive feedback, promotional blurbs, and reviews: Raymond Hillis, Edgar Barnett, Ernest Hartmann, and Jacqueline Sallade. At UCLA 40 years ago my roommate, Ray Hillis, majored in psychology. Eventually I followed his footsteps—thank you Ray.

Too, I thank Anees Sheikh, The *Imagery and Human Development Series* Editor of Baywood, for his support in this project, and Bobbi Olszewski and Joi Tamber-Brooks for their work in editing and promoting this book.

Beowulf, though written in Old English, is a Viking-Icelandic story. While writing this book, with the excitement of my personal discovery of the Icelandic Sagas, I frequently thought of a neighbor of 20 plus years ago, Michael Bell, now of the University of Colorado. With fond curiosity I remember Mike because of his doctorate in the esoteric field of Icelandic Literature. I was pleased when he agreed to write the Foreword.

A neighbor in his youth and now a citizen of the world is Benjamin Ruhe, the artist-illustrator for this book. I have greatly enjoyed watching Ben's art develop over the years and offer a special thanks to him.

CHAPTER I

The Imagery of Dreams, Hypnosis, and Myth

DREAMS

A dream commonly causes great internal commotion. Its bizarre nature opens the dreamer to many questions. "Where did the dream come from?" "What does it mean?" "Is it going to happen?" The dreamer is often eager to talk about the dream and somehow knows the dream is important. Dreams are not random and meaningless. The emotional reactions to dreams—the anxiety, fatigue, and excitement—only add to our belief that dreams must be important. Dreams are created in our unconscious mind. Understanding the meaning of dreams can open doors to real change in the course of psychotherapy.

Consider a dream of 27-year-old Mandi: "I'm waiting in a checkout line of a market with only a half gallon of milk. Several people are in front of me in line. The woman next in front of me is older, probably in her fifties. I've a great urge to give her a shove. Several people are in front of her, I think maybe another woman and two men. It's the express line. Each is carrying only a couple of things. I've had this dream many times until a couple of months ago, when I dreamt I actually pushed this woman that was in front of me. I woke up and don't remember what happened after that, but I haven't had the dream since."

Dreams provide messages from the unconscious mind, as do the images produced in hypnotic trance. These messages may tell of internal struggles and emotional pain that parallel the trauma or emotionally painful family behaviors and attitudes that affect and limit the dreamer's life. The purpose of this book about psychotherapy is to present ways to make sense of these unconscious messages and to use these messages to facilitate personal understanding and internal or unconscious change. Mandi may attempt to change using will power, but real change occurs only when internal or unconscious self-images change. As we shall see, helping Mandi find meaning in her dream is one step in her journey to health. Beginning with Chapter IV, the six individuals studied in this book will be led, first, to identify the incidents of abuse and/or emotionally painful family behaviors and attitudes that affected and limited their lives. Then, hypnotic and dream work strategies will be offered to help these individuals free themselves from these limits.

I asked Mandi to tell me more about the feelings of the Mandi in her dream who had the urge to push the woman in the checkout line. She answered, "I was horrified by the urge but thought it would be fun, too—funny, hilariously funny—watching one person fall into the next, watching the horror and amazement on their faces as they each fell. I couldn't help but laugh inside at what they would think. How outrageous."

A Gestalt dream work technique of Fritz Perls (1970) is used to help the client identify with each part of a dream. Identifying with each part of the dream helps the client understand the unconscious processes. I suggested to Mandi, "Consider these two parts of you separately and find them inside of you. One part is horrified about doing something so outrageous. The other part of you finds such an outrageous act hilariously funny and could enjoy the amazement of others. Find each of those parts within you. What do you find?"

Mandi, who is moderately obese, laughs, "I have sat and eaten a whole half gallon of ice cream at one time and had the thought of how horrified people would be, how horrified my mother would be, to see me eat it."

I continued, "Take these feelings even further back into your childhood. Can you find them there?"

Mandi had been in weekly sessions of therapy for about a month and was somewhat experienced in dream work and hypnosis. She came to therapy because of problems she had with her adolescent daughter, but the focus of attention quickly shifted to personal issues, issues that did affect her daughter. After a minute's thought, she answered. "Sure, my mother was often outraged about things I would do, about what I would want to wear to school like a short skirt on a snowy day. She would always say, 'What would other people think?' I hate it when she says that. I was a good kid. I hardly ever did anything to upset my mother except wearing outrageous things to school. I was very responsible. I did well in school. I did chores around the house, but I rebelled by wearing bizarre things to school. I hated hearing 'what would other people think?'" Though her mother's comments may have been the mother's way of showing she loved and cared for Mandi, to Mandi these comments were judgmental and critical. Mandi was wounded repeatedly by these comments, which she heard as conditional love. As innocent as these family attitudes and behaviors may be, the wounds caused do affect and limit one's life and are passed on from generation to generation.

HYPNOSIS

A variety of hypnotic guided imagery techniques can also provide direct access to the unconscious and can be used in the same manner as dreams.

I suggested to Mandi, "Sit back and relax." After I led her through a hypnotic induction for relaxation, I asked her, "Take the feeling you feel when you think of doing something outrageous, take this feeling back through time. Watch your life go by—people, places, events, holidays, seasons—be curious and wondering as you go back through time, carrying this feeling with you. As you go back through time, carrying this feeling, something will soon catch your attention. When it does, lift the index finger of your left hand." She lifted her finger. "Tell me what is happening."

"I'm about to leave the house for school. I'm wearing jeans with the knees ripped and a hole in the butt. I look in the mirror and can see the red from my panties through the hole. I laugh when I see it, know my mother is going to freak, but I don't care. . . . My mother is yelling, 'What are your teachers going to think?' I just yell back, 'I'm late for school' and run out the door."

"What is happening now?"

"I'm walking down the street and meet one of my girl friends. I turn and show her the hole. She puts her hand over her mouth and laughs."

"How do you feel? Let your adult self go back and be with your teenage self and let your adult self help your younger self find the best words to describe how you feel."

"I feel excited. I'm laughing and feel carefree."

"Go back for a minute to just before you left the house. Your mother is saying 'what are other people going to think?' What do you feel?"

"I feel angry, defiant, like I'd like to stick my tongue out at her. I hate when she says 'what will other people think?' I'd never say it to my kids."

"Now, let your adult self go back and be with your younger self. Help your younger self find the right words to tell your mom what you need from her."

"I know what you're asking, but this time I'm sort of happy she said it because it gave me an excuse to run out the door. I'll try to think of some other times . . . Yeah, 'Mom, I need you to let me be me, to let me know you understand my feelings.'"

Mandi was familiar with this procedure. During an earlier session we had talked about the healing nature of stating what one needs from one's mother (or father), about how such statements tell one how one wants to be. Saying, "I will never say 'What will other people think?'" tells one nothing about the alternatives of how one wants to be or what one could say.

Though the phrase "what will other people think" is not what most people would consider abusive, it was a major determinant of Mandi's defiant behaviors. She let it limit her freedom in such endeavors as losing weight. For Mandi, this phrase needed to be considered significant in the healing process, a process that could eventually allow Mandi greater freedom to make decisions in her life.

To reiterate, the purpose of this book is to examine ways to access the unconscious mind through dreams and hypnosis, to identify incidents of abuse and/or family behaviors and attitudes that affect and limit one's life, and to understand the process of healing—of freeing oneself from these limits. The unconscious processes of an individual in the process of healing are extremely personal and unique, yet each of us has the capacity to understand these experiences of others. We are able to empathize because we have had similar experiences. There exists among the people of a group, if not all people, in common unconscious processes that allow such empathy. These group unconscious processes allow us to generalize from one person to another. How can we access the unconscious processes in common to all people, at least for the people of a particular cultural group? The collected myth of the group offers us this understanding of the in common unconscious processes.

MYTH

Whereas dreams, guided imagery, and hypnosis provide an understanding of unconscious processes at an individual level, myths offer a more global understanding of the functioning of the unconscious mind in the process of healing. Ancient myths can be considered the dreams of our ancestors. Myths have been refined over the years to provide this global understanding. Ancient myths can be understood at their deepest level using the same techniques of dream work as offered through Gestalt Therapy. Jung suggests we need to examine a series of dreams rather than a single dream to understand the unconscious process. Ancient myths are equivalent to a series of dreams and are stories to which we can all relate through our unconscious mind.

One particular myth, the old English myth of Beowulf, offers us a map of a journey through the unconscious mind to overcome and heal the wounds of childhood trauma and emotionally painful family behaviors and attitudes. As you may recall if you read this myth in school, the story begins with Scyld Scefing as an infant, abandoned on the shores of Denmark. This infant grows to become the first great king of the Danes. His son, grandson, and great grandson, each in their turn, become even greater kings than their father. Our story is about the great King Hrothgar, the great grandson of Scyld Scefing.

Each chapter of this book will examine a section of this story to provide us with greater understanding of the healing process. Each part of a dream or myth, each element and person, can be found within each of us. This introduction to King Hrothgar offers us an example of dissociation. Scyld Scefing represents that early part of us who was abandoned or traumatized in some way. Yet, just as King Hrothgar is separated or dissociated from the trauma by three generations, the part of us in the present does not remember or is dissociated from the trauma.

The trauma of Scyld Scefing is very much alive in King Hrothgar, as we will see. Though this great and benevolent king is loved by his people, a great tormentor destroys his will and strength. Each night, Grendel, a powerful and evil monster, comes into the King's great banquet hall and kills one or more of his men. For twelve years, the people of Denmark have had to hide from this monster to protect their lives. So far, no warrior has been strong enough to rid the kingdom of Grendel.

In our lives we have such tormentors: fears, anxieties, obsessions, depression, marital discord, bad habits, etc. These tormentors limit our lives and prevent us from living comfortably and effectively. We may live for years believing we lack the ability to conquer these tormentors with our usual and ineffective defenses. As we shall see, our usual defenses and beliefs can actually strengthen our tormentor, just as Grendel's continued slaughter provides him with greater self-confidence. We will need to find new ways to fight our tormentors.

Chapters II and III, which examine the historic factors that prepare a client for therapy, correspond to this first, historic portion of the Beowulf myth. Therapy to overcome one's tormentor begins in Chapter IV when Beowulf, our powerful inner warrior, enters the story. Beowulf has heard, from his home across the sea, of the plight of King Hrothgar and takes on the challenge to rid this King of the Danes of his torment by killing Grendel. As the story progresses, after Beowulf arrives and after the evening festivities end, Beowulf and his men bed down in the great hall of the king to await Grendel. When Grendel enters, Beowulf lies naked, pretending to be asleep. Beowulf rises, grabs hold of Grendel's arm, and refuses to let go. After a violent struggle Grendel pulls away, leaving his arm behind. Like Hrothgar's hero, our own inner Beowulf comes to us when we least expect him, from our unconscious mind, and uses a weapon we would least expect, his bare hands. Our usual defenses are ineffective and interfere with our natural inner, bare handed strength.

If we abandon our defenses and trust our inherent strength, we can win in the battle over our tormentor. We have the ability to overcome our tormentor by facing it without our defenses, facing it naked and refusing to let go. When we do so, our tormentor loses strength and dies. We then celebrate our victory as King Hrothgar, Beowulf, and their retainers celebrate.

But that night, as the celebration ends and the celebrants fall asleep, Grendel's mother enters to seek revenge for her son's death, attacking and killing one of the Geat warriors. Likewise, overcoming our tormentor opens the door to the deeper problem: the real tormentor, our trauma or painful family behaviors and attitudes, hidden deep in the murky lake of our unconscious. With our victory over Grendel, we are now prepared to face this greater, original tormentor, the mother of Grendel.

Beowulf tracks Grendel's mother to a lake seething with blood and monsters. Wearing his armor, he dives in and fights his way to the bottom. At the bottom, Grendel's mother finds him and takes him to her cave, where they begin their fight to the death. Although she is unable to penetrate his armor, Beowulf's own weapons cannot stop his adversary. He then discovers in her lair a famous sword made by giants, a sword an ordinary man would be unable to lift. Beowulf swings this sword and severs the neck of Grendel's mother, and in death, her fiery blood dissolves the sword.

To find the origin of our torment—the trauma of our childhood—we need to track it down to its source, at the bottom of a murky lake, deep within our unconscious. When we find it, we must face it with all our strength. We have collected much armor, our many defenses, from our lifelong but unconscious battle to deal with this torment. These defenses continue to be effective but lead us to the usual stalemate—otherwise our tormentor already would be dead. For victory, we need to uncover and understand our tormentor's strength—the giant's sword—and use it against her (or him). Only then can we conquer the effect the trauma has had on us. We cut off the monster's head, i.e., cut off the effect the trauma had on us, and carry signs of our victory to the surface of the lake, back home to the great hall of King Hrothgar. Only then are we truly able to celebrate. This myth of Beowulf offers us an understanding of the unconscious process of healing and a recipe for the necessary ingredients to attain a new sense of freedom in life.

This story of Hrothgar, Beowulf, and Grendel and his mother will now be retold in detail, interspersed with clinical examples from my experiences in therapy. Following the outline of the myth, Chapter II presents the development of the emotional problems of despairing individuals who will eventually seek therapy. Chapter III examines how the despair leads individuals to seek help. Chapter IV and the remaining chapters examine the course of therapy for six people. Following the course of therapy from beginning to end brings us around full circle, resolving the problem developed in Chapters II and III.

CHAPTER II

The Lineage of Hrothgar: Dissociation from Trauma

The story of the great Geat warrior Beowulf opens by tracing the ancestry of Hrothgar, king of the Danes. Hrothgar's great-grandfather, Scyld Scefing, survives as an infant castaway on the shores of Denmark. Without knowledge of his heritage he grows to conquer nations and collect tribute from his neighbors to become the first great king of Denmark. Scyld Scefing's son, Beowulf, not the great Geat warrior and hero of our story, was born to become the second king of Denmark. King Beowulf's son, Healfdene, became the third great king. Finally, Hrothgar, the son of Healfdene, was born to become the fourth and greatest king of the four.

As we develop and dissociate from the pain of our early abandonment or trauma, we grow through three stages of greater dissociation. As we grow in strength, our inner king strives to become a healthy and loved king. As we grow through our first and earliest infant stage, we learn to survive our trauma. This first stage is represented by Scyld Scefing. We then grow in self confidence during our childhood, depicted by King Beowulf, and adolescence, represented by Healfdene. We finally attain adulthood as portrayed by Hrothgar. Growth through these four developmental stages, Scyld Scefing, Beowulf, Healfdene, and Hrothgar, provide us with the strength we need to eventually heal the trauma of our infancy.

Returning to the earliest infant stage, after he is abandoned, Scyld Scefing grows to conquer nations and exact tribute from his neighbors. Although his parents, as often happens, have had little control over his fate, nevertheless Scyld Scefing experienced being abandoned. Abandonment is one kind of trauma, and an infantile temper tantrum is one way to exact tribute from our neighbors. Temper tantrums provide us with distraction from and numb our pain of abandonment. Other kinds of trauma—physical, sexual, and emotional—and other forms of exacting tribute begin to develop early in infancy and childhood. Tribute may be exacted with defiance, dependency, passivity, anxiety, depression, obsessions, phobias, and an infinite number of acting out behaviors. Each means of exacting tribute offers us a way to numb the pain of trauma and collect from others what we believe is due us.

Scyld Scefing's son Beowulf, by his goodness and generous gifts, becomes a most loved king of the people of Denmark. (The reader may find confusion in two characters with the same name and is again reminded that this King Beowulf, the son of Scyld Scefing, is not the warrior Beowulf, the hero and protector of Hrothgar.) As we grow from infancy into our early childhood years, we learn to get our own way by finding both healthy and unhealthy ways to please others. We smile and coo. We make noises that eventually take the form of understandable words, and we learn many other ways to please.

When death approaches, Scyld Scefing is set to sea surrounded with wealth. When we have learned to gain love through benevolence, we then deny, ignore, or dissociate from the earlier life of abandonment, temper tantrums, and tyranny. Our earlier life dies, the death of the oldest self, Scyld Scefing.

We have now forgotten the pain of the original trauma or painful family behaviors and attitudes and find security in the power of benevolence. We do those things that please others and receive love in return. In the security of this regal family, the high-minded Healfdene, the third generation, is born. Healfdene is a fierce patriarch who finds security in forming an army. He establishes relationships with neighbors, develops a strong base of power to raise his family, and becomes most effective in life.

Finally, Healfdene's son, Hrothgar, the fourth generation, becomes established and builds the large hall, Heorot, as a secure center for his kingdom. The old English word "Heorot" can be translated "hart" or stag, a deer fleet of foot, swift and free. Hrothgar values the security of Heorot and finds within it a new sense of freedom, the freedom of this swift and free animal. Yet a deer knows that danger lurks nearby. Only with this great security and a new sense of freedom is Hrothgar prepared to face the painful trauma of his dissociated infancy, an infancy wrought with nearby danger and emotional pain. Thus enters the scene the monster Grendel.

The process of dissociation, which provides us with increasing security and strength, allows us to eventually face the pain of childhood's loneliness and desertion. This common pattern prepares us to face our tormentor of the present, Grendel, and opens the door for psychotherapy and change.

THE NATURE OF TRAUMA

When abuse is mentioned, we think first of physical and sexual abuse, the kinds of abuse frequently documented in newspapers. Such trauma is real and a problem in our society. Another kind of trauma is desertion or abandonment. We occasionally read of parents who leave for short trips or vacations, leaving their young children home alone. We think of single mothers who need to work and find they have no other alternative than to leave their children home alone or alone to roam a shopping mall. This trauma is also real and important to this story. Yet the real trauma of separation, some therapists believe, originates in our initial separation from the womb. Everyone experiences the original trauma of exiting their prenatal place of warmth and comfort and entering a world of pain and chaos. We as good parents may be aware of these more obvious forms of trauma, but we are generally unaware of the more subtle feelings of loneliness and desertion experienced by our children in our insensitivity to them. Alice Miller (1981) reflects: "sometimes I ask myself whether it will ever be possible for us to grasp the extent of the loneliness and desertion to which we were exposed as children, and, hence, intrapsychically still are exposed as adults."

As good, loving parents, we know what is best for our children. We offer them our advice. We assure them that their worries, their hurts, their disappointments are insignificant in the light of their future. We give our word their future life will make their present problems seem minute. But in doing so, we diminish what is important to our children. This discounting of our children's feelings alone can provide our children with a formidable sense of loneliness.

I sat on the floor one afternoon with five-year-old Brad, a boy small for his kindergarten class, both in age and stature. Brad's mother sat on the couch watching us in play therapy. After a few minutes of play, Brad began telling me about how another boy cut in front of him in line for the drinking fountain.

"That must have hurt your feelings," I said.

"Yes, I was so mad. He was big and he scared me."

"He could have hurt you."

In a few moments, his hands left the Lego blocks and he told me how he hated school because he was the smallest boy in the class.

At the end of the play his mother commented, "I didn't realize how bad he felt. He had told me about the line to the drinking fountain and I told him to not worry, he would get big." How lonely Brad must have felt.

Beyond the tendency to diminish our children's feelings, we, as parents, with the best intent, become involved, sometimes excessively, in our children's activities and achievements, if those activities and achievements meet with our approval. We are excited about our children's performance at recitals when we pay for lessons. Sport buffs cheer their children from the stands. We become thrilled by their good grades and fretful when grades are poor.

One young adult in therapy recalled playing goalie for his youth's soccer team. Louie heard the voice of his mother, his number one fan, screaming for him above all others from the bleachers. He walked off the field and refused to play again. As an adult he finally found the words: "The game was more important to my mother than to me. I felt ripped off. She stole it from me." How lonely he must have felt—loneliness escalated by his inability to express himself, to put into words a reasonable explanation of why he needed to walk off the field.

We have our values, manners we cherish, ideas, and beliefs we want for our children. We want to protect our children from making the mistakes we made in our childhood. We become preoccupied in teaching, moralizing, and forcing these values and beliefs on our children. Again, our children's beliefs, their own chance to learn from experience, their own needs and values are diminished, ignored, and forgotten. Thus, the world of our children can be a world of intense loneliness and desertion.

We, as good parents, worry about children who suffer from physical and sexual abuse. Such suffering is horrendous, but even the best of us continue to ignore our own children's feelings and pressure our children to be as we want. We are over-involved in what is important to us and forget to pay attention to what is important to our child. Our children suffer, but since we appear to be such great parents, this suffering is not understood by our children. Children do not have the sophisticated language to put their suffering into words. Parents, grandparents, teachers, and other important adults are "gods" to the child, praising the child's strengths but lacking awareness of the child's suffering. Children do not have a chance to put their feelings into words even if they had command of those words. They are not afforded the chance to understand their feelings. They stand alone, deserted.

You might be saying I am overstating the suffering and pain of childhood. You might feel this is an unnecessary guilt trip since your children, and most children, survive, excel, and are happy. They laugh and play. They run to our arms. They hug us and love us. They are carefree. Children are tremendously resilient, often apparently unfazed by such insensitivities, hurts, or disappointments. But as a psychologist, I work with children who are now adults—adults who are intra-psychically still exposed to the emptiness and desertion of their childhood. Most of these adults begin therapy praising their parents, yet behind the problems they present in therapy are feelings of emptiness, loneliness, and abandonment, feelings we will eventually name as Grendel's mother.

THE FIRST GENERATION: EXACTING TRIBUTE

As he grows in strength, Scyld Scefing strikes terror in the hearts of his neighbors. He exacts obedience and tribute from the people of every land.

Children of abuse, of loneliness and desertion, find many ways to cope, to survive. They may act out with temper tantrums. They may pull back and find power in their fantasies. They may dream of getting even or they may find real ways of getting even, some ways more constructive than others. They may excel in school to escape, or they may fail. In each case they cause their parents to react or worry, exacting tribute from them, though when the child excels in school to escape, the tribute may not be collected until later in life in the form of behavioral, emotional, and thought disorders.

The story indicates that, before Scyld Scefing, the people had been kingless, there had been misery and chaos, and God sent this king to comfort the people. Before our children gain the strength of their inner tyrant king, they feel hopeless and empty, they feel the pain and chaos of their initial separation from the womb. From these unbearable feelings the tyrant king is born. Scyld Scefing "finds consolation for this misfortune" of abandonment and loneliness by becoming the tyrant king.

Craig, a successful management-level 45 year old, came to therapy for anxiety and obsessive worry. He recalled how his mother used to say to his younger brother, "Why can't you be like Craig?" How many good parents use this phrase? What could be wrong with it? After all, Craig should be proud of his good behavior and feel the love and support due him from his mother. He then and even now did not understand his resentment, the anger he felt when he heard those words from his mother.

Craig eventually found his own words: "To please mom I had to be perfect; I had a lot to live up to. I couldn't be just a six-year-old boy." He continues, "My younger brother always resented me. Mom put me in between. Keith blamed me. I missed out on having a brother with whom I was close."

How can we expect a young boy to understand this bind, a bind that drives him to excel, to be a type-A perfectionist, to conquer the world and exact tribute?

When tribute is exacted, we first think of it as being exacted on our "overseas neighbors"—our parents or teachers. But Craig exacted tribute, his obsessive worry, on his own warrior self, that part of him that sets goals and goes after them. He became his own worst enemy. The tribute exacted is in the long run on ourselves, on the parent archetype within us, though it may also be on our parents.

The parents of a five-year-old boy came to therapy because of their son's unruly and defiant behavior. Sammy would hit his mother and pull her hair when it was within reach. He would run out of the house, refusing to stop when ordered to do so. He could not be trusted around his younger sister. The parents were at wits' end. Mom would scream. She would cry. She might try to set Sammy on a chair or send him to his room, but he would not stay. She felt powerless. She was powerless. Sammy had power over her to upset her. He had control of her. He could make her scream. He could make her cry.

A parent is a child's first understanding of God. God is supposed to be omnipotent. But mom did not show the omnipotent, steadfast stability and strength of God. Instead, Sammy had the power of God over his mother, but he had neither the maturity nor the security to have this power. Although the cause was too abstract for a five year old to comprehend, Sammy was acting out of insecurity, fear, and resentment. Parental authority is the only strength a child knows. When loving firmness vanishes into parental fear and powerlessness, the children stand in a vacuum of insecurity and panic. In order for the parent to regain needed parental authority, therapy for the parent would seem more appropriate than therapy for the child. One purpose of this book is to demonstrate how adults can be helped on their life's journey to surmount their own trauma and insecurity and to become secure and loving spouses and/or parents. Therapy needs to teach parents security and loving firmness.

Another client, Megan, recalled her father's maxim: "If you have nothing important to say, say nothing at all." Only in therapy did she realize the bind caused by this phrase. She dearly wanted to be close to her father, and to do so, she had to keep an emotional distance, because to him, emotional expression was not important. We sadly laughed at the thought that seeing a dead skunk in the middle of the road is something important, whereas hurt feelings are unimportant. Megan grew up feeling very empty in her relationship with her father, and now she felt empty with her husband, expecting him also to prefer emotional distance rather than closeness in their relationship. Tribute was exacted on her nurturing self and, outwardly, on her husband.

These patterns of response to trauma are carried into adult life, becoming the currency of our tribute. We know no other way to react in life even though our patterns of reaction are pain-inducing, exacting great personal toll or tribute. A variety of these patterns became evident with a group of survivors of abuse. Seven people entered group therapy, each with a different currency of tribute. One came with frequent panic or anxiety attacks. She recalled lying in bed, feeling terror when her parents fought. A second tended to "space out" in fantasy at inopportune times. She recalled wishing she had some magical powers she could use to rescue her when abused by her father. A third suffered from depression and a sense of emptiness. She remembered denying her own needs, wishing to do everything she could do to please her foster family after her parents abandoned her. She felt empty while doing all she could to please her husband. A fourth would explode in rage after an incident of parental sex abuse, a rage directed at her mother, siblings, or others in her life, and, from their perspective, for no apparent reason. She continues to rage in her marriage. A fifth was a worrier, just as her mother was a worrier.

The sixth is jealous and fears her husband is having an extramarital affair. She is now aware of how she has never trusted men. In her adolescence she could not stay in a relationship because of her jealousy, believing each boyfriend was unfaithful, just as her father had been unfaithful to her mother. Her parents' divorce was very painful because, until then, she had trusted her father and was close to him. Her mother was never available to her. In this divorce, she didn't know to whom to turn, which way to go.

The seventh member explodes in rage at her own imperfections, as well as the imperfections of her husband and children. Explosive rage is typical type A personality behavior. She could never please her successful, critical, and demanding father no matter how hard she tried to succeed. At these earlier points in life's process, the currencies of tribute were being defined. For all of us, we were not aware of the problems that lay ahead. In the following chapters, we will explore the process of uncovery and change, of becoming aware of our currencies of tribute and finding new ways to live and be.

THE SECOND GENERATION: SEEKING TO PLEASE

God grants Scyld Scefing a son, Beowulf (not the warrior-slayer of Grendel). This prince is protected by his father the king and becomes renowned for his goodness and generous gifts. These qualities bring him the support of many retainers and people who remain loyal in the time of war. Through his actions he earns praise and prospers.

What part of us is this Beowulf, the grandfather to Hrothgar? We have grown beyond the demanding nature of infancy and are beginning to realize that we need to be kind and generous in order to have friends. A child who is loved learns to love. Yet Beowulf is the offspring of the trauma of abandonment. He fits well the definition of the narcissist who seeks to manipulate others to find security and love in material things, as described by John Bowlby (Masterson, 1988). Bowlby studied hospitalized children 32 months old or younger who had to deal with an abrupt change in their life, usually the loss of an ever-present mother. He found that for many of these children, the child, after a period of showing acute distress at having lost its mother, gave up trust and affection for a mothering figure, whether mother or nurse. The child then became "increasingly self-centered and, instead of having desires and feelings toward people, he became preoccupied with material things that wouldn't let him down. . . . The child became more interested in the presents a parent or nurse might bring than in the parent or nurse as people." With feelings of abandonment, this child may find some satisfaction in amassing tribute but as he grows he will learn that he can buy loyalty, as false as it may be, with his newly gained wealth.

One client in therapy recalled, from his youth, his one claim to fame. Carl was the only boy among his friends who had a job. He felt great spending the money he earned on his friends. Now, he realizes he does not trust his friends because they are only there for his money. His main goal in life, since his youth, has been to provide well for his wife and children. Now he feels very alienated from them, believing they are simply taking advantage of him. Despair has taken over his life. Initially in therapy there was no recognition of childhood trauma. Later Carl was able to describe how his parents spent long hours in the store they owned and showed irritation if he sought their attention. He was able to admit he felt abandoned by his parents but found some satisfaction in the attention he received from his friends when buying their friendship.

I recall a young woman who had recently been married. What Mae did as a child who had been placed in a foster home she now was doing with her husband. From the first day she was placed in a foster home she worked hard to please her foster parents, to earn their love. This work included washing dishes, doing the laundry, cleaning, and cooking when she was allowed. Mae was also a good student in school. She was driven beyond reason to be the perfect child. When she continued to be as driven in her married life to win her husband's love, problems began to develop. Her husband wanted her to slow down and to enjoy life and their relationship. Mark felt he did not know her. He wanted some of her time. Unlike the woman in the group who, as a foster-child, tried to please, Mae's husband did not take advantage of the situation.

Because of their feelings of alienation, these clients are driven to recoup love by seeking to please others. Unlike the knight-errant or the philanthropist, whose altruistic behavior is motivated by an inherent desire to do good for others, the people pleaser is motivated by an inner feeling of emptiness. Whereas the altruist exhibits a self-identity separate from giving, people pleasers lose their identity in their need to please. Unlike the placater or appeaser whose behavior is motivated by a fear of negative emotional expression and a need to avoid discomfort, people pleasers seek comfort in making others happy. Unlike the sycophant, the fawner whose neediness is most apparent and whose obsequious actions cause others to feel uncomfortable, the people pleaser's behavior is appreciated and neediness is not apparent.

The rules of good etiquette, when applied diligently, offer a way to please others. By adhering to these rules a person seeks to make the other comfortable. These rules are defined by the culture and are especially refined in the English culture. Carol Tavris (1982) holds the belief that the manner in which people deal with anger is culturally defined and that the English avoid the expression of anger through the many rules of etiquette. Adhering to these rules, each individual seeks to make others comfortable and eliminate the place for anger. Such individuals learn not to experience anger or resentment but hold a primary goal of seeking to make others comfortable. Adhering to these rules may be motivated by a person's set of values, as in the knight-errant, or by one's need to please.

Can individuals please others in a spontaneous, natural way? People who have been truly loved feel a sense of self-confidence and trust. These people are spontaneous and natural in loving and relating to others. These natural loving people feel they have considerable control over their lives and their environment. They accurately trust their own judgment in relating to others. As they grew, these individuals were trusted in a loving manner. Their parents had confidence in them appropriate to their stages of development. When they were infants, their parents changed their diapers in a loving manner, accepting the dirty diaper as a natural act of infancy. The development of a child physically, emotionally, intellectually, and spiritually, is natural, can be trusted to occur, and is amazing to observe. No matter what a child's mental capacity, as the child grows, development can be appreciated with a parental attitude of amazement and trust.

If, as parents, we could maintain an attitude of trust, awe and reverence for our children, they could not help but grow with trust, self-confidence, and a natural ability to love. The effect of holding such an attitude is quickly seen in the ancient stories of most cultures, e.g., the Celtic story of Cuchulain of Muirthemne and the biblical story of the birth of Jesus. Imagine if an angel came down and told you as a parent that your child was special, divine, and a child of God. Imagine the effect this would have on your attitude in raising your children. The lives of these children in the ancient writings were truly amazing.

Dorothy Cantor (1992) interviewed 25 high-ranking woman politicians, asking them about the messages they received from their parents as children. These messages were summarized:

- You are loved and special!
- You can set goals and do anything you want!
- It is permissible to take risks!
- You can use and enjoy creative aggression which allows you to set a goal and go after it!
- You can dream of greatness!

With such childhood messages, we each would have the spontaneous love, confidence, and the trust in our own judgment to become benevolent leaders. We would experience divinity within us. Yet for many of us, the king within has experienced abandonment and the trauma of childhood. This book is about those of us who have lost this sense of divinity.

THE DEATH OF SCYLD: THE TIME FOR DISSOCIATION

After a long reign as king, Scyld's hour comes and his dearest retainers carry their beloved leader to the shore. A royal vessel is prepared with great treasures gained from ventures into distant lands. The king's body is placed midship and sadly sent to sea. "No one can say who receives this impressive cargo."

The pained part of us, pained because of our abandonment, dies and is sent to sea. This death is our dissociation from this pain. The clearest examples of dissociation may be from the survivors of incest. These survivors typically report, "I saw myself lying on the bed as if I were watching from the far corner of the room." One woman recalled, "For a number of years I thought it was the bogeyman until one day I opened my eyes to see it was my stepfather." Dissociation is the experience of "it is really not happening to me" or "what is happening is really not what it is." One man recalled being beaten as a child: "I was Superman. I stood there smiling because I could not feel a thing. It proved I was really Superman."

Dissociation can be experienced with a sense of power, like that of Superman or of the great warrior, Scyld Scefing. As with this warrior, a part of the traumatized person dies and is set adrift. The power to dissociate is great and quickly becomes a relied upon way of avoiding any physical or emotional pain throughout life no matter how minor. The woman in the group who fantasized magical powers to deal with her abusing father found fantasizing an easy way to avoid the daily pressures at work, to the point that this dissociation affected her job performance and her job was in jeopardy.

A child's lack of vocabulary to describe feelings or what is happening aids the child in the denial of or dissociation from trauma. Letting feelings and thoughts die, setting them adrift at sea, is facilitated by a child's lack of words to describe the experiences of abuse. So often in therapy the word "it" is used to describe the occurrence of incest or other form of abuse. On occasion the child may invent a new language. On one occasion the woman referred to the incidents of incest as "he freezed me," watching herself lying motionless from the corner of the room. Dissociation for this woman takes the form of sitting motionless as if in a catatonic state.

A child's lack of abstract reasoning also supports the tendency to dissociate. In the act of incest, the abuser's excitement, heavy breathing, fear or guilt, or words of justification, e.g., "I love you," or "I'm not going to hurt you" are unexplainable in a child's way of concrete reasoning. One young adult, Bonnie, realized she was afraid of being around her grandfather but did not know why. During a session of hypnotic time regression, she relived an incident when she was three years old. Bonnie was staying with her grandmother who was giving her a bath. The grandmother was called to the telephone and while on the phone, the grandfather came into the bathroom. He announced, "I am not going to hurt you" while supposedly continuing with the bath. The implication of this phrase is "I am hurting you" or "you should be expecting me to hurt you." Even though he may not have physically hurt her, the phrase implied some other motivation the three year old did not have the reasoning ability to understand. The phrase frightened her for some unexplainable reason.

These abused individuals typically do whatever they can to please the abuser: "I tried to do everything I could to please Dad. I never complained. If I could make Dad happy, maybe he would not do 'it' to me." Beowulf, the son of Scyld Scefing, lived beyond his father as a benevolent and kind king, seeking to please his people. Thus did King Beowulf live with the trauma of abandonment, although it did not consciously affect his life. To perfect dissociation from trauma, a person needs continually to deny the trauma and replace it with a good life, real or imaginary. What better way to attain a good life than to work to please others without complaint. With the good life that results from pleasing others, a person really begins to forget about the trauma.

As life continues, the traumatized child finds continued strength in pleasing others—in becoming a powerful warrior in quest of success, academically, athletically, religiously, socially, and/or sexually, attaining one victory after another. These victories are ways of escaping the trauma, of escaping the family, and of feeling loved by teachers, coaches, pillars of the church, or successive lovers. With each victory, the trauma vanishes further into the fog at sea.

The completeness of this forgetting is sometimes incredible. Clients come to therapy with such comments as "I had a dream of being raped but I don't think I was ever raped," or "I have this strange feeling something terrible happened to me when I was five," or "I can't remember anything between when I was three and seven." Often clients come to therapy for other emotional problems with no clue or memory of any abuse or incest. Only while dealing with the auxiliary emotional problem does the memory of the abuse begin to arise. The memory had been sent to sea, lost in the fog, but usually the skeleton returns to shore. The process of finding, surmounting, and healing these skeletons or wounds is the topic of this book.

Peggy repeatedly had an image of a darkened room and a disheveled bed that would trigger a sense of panic. She could not remember living in a house with this room and bed. Nanna had a dream of being a golf caddie for her father. When she reached into the golf bag to pull out a club, she found she was pulling on his penis. Craig was obsessed about making mistakes at work. He checked and double checked his work fearing he might unknowingly write something that would offend someone or intentionally, but without remembering, make a mistake. He would eventually be able to express his anger at his mother, father, and grandfather, each of whom tormented him in a different way. Meanwhile, his obsessive worry was his way of protecting himself from his anger.

A woman diagnosed as schizophrenic and hospitalized showed a severe muscle tic, twisting her head and neck, reminiscent of the way a person would twist their head when hit in the side of the head. While in therapy, Anabel would talk in a very grandiose manner, never about her family, but about her future. One day, just on a whim, I brought a broom into the therapy room and laid it against one of the chairs. On this day, Anabel's neck twists greatly increased and she rambled on, still in a grandiose manner—about her mother. Her grandiose manner may have been a sign of her dissociation from the abuse of being hit with a broom. Grandiosity is a common way of covering up the pain of trauma and what can be more grandiose than becoming a powerful and wealthy king.

THE THIRD GENERATION: THE PAYOFF OF SUCCESS

Eventually the great Healfdene, son of Beowulf, is born. In his turn, he rules Denmark as a fierce warrior and king. Healfdene's supportive followers gather by him because of his benevolence and provide him with great strength. This next stage of life, represented by Healfdene, has the strength of a great and fierce king with a great number of retainers. Similarly, in our youth we grow in power, as we gain "retainers" internally by demonstrating deeds of strength and benevolence and developing skills in which we are confident. We begin to gain a sense of control over our actions and our environment. This young adult stage of development is the time we begin on the real journey toward success, power, and fame, gaining omnipotence in our ability to accomplish any goals we may set for ourselves. Youths typically believe they know everything. Only with greater maturity do we realize there is much more to learn.

This young adult stage provides us with a sense of self-importance that allows us to put our trauma in the distant past and to forget it. The sense of being abandoned or traumatized has long been repressed and is no longer in our conscious thoughts. The remainder of this poem of Beowulf is about regaining and dealing with this lost knowledge.

As we proceed in a chosen direction in life, the warrior energy within us grows. It is an energy that is directed and single minded. This energy may be positive and lead us to socially acceptable activities, such as going to college or beginning in a career. Or this energy may be negative, leading us into drugs, gang activities, and crime. The goals and activities are pursued, sometimes effectively, sometimes ineffectively. Derived from our repressed feelings of the pain from trauma and a need to escape this pain, the warrior energy is great, possibly leading us into the frenzied activities of the type-A personality. Or, in the case of rebellion against socially acceptable norms, we may demonstrate equally intense energy in our antisocial acts.

Though he is fierce, Healfdene still has the knowledge of how to treat his allies, his retainers. The knowledge or need to be good and generous is in his blood, inherited from his father. It is not just with money that he retains his friends; now he can impress them with his strength and power. But are they really his friends? Are his "friends" just going along for the ride to get what they can? Are they his friends by intimidation? These nagging questions continue to live within. "Since my parents (great grandparents) did not love me and abandoned me, why should anyone really love me?" This question is so frequently repeated in therapy. For the person having an extramarital affair: "if every person on this earth loved me, was willing to have sex with me, it still would not be enough. I need to love myself first." The continued nagging sense of emptiness, the void, provides the impetus for the warrior energy.

Charlene, a high achieving professional woman, described her father as emotionally distant. He was in high level management of a large business, and a driven man. She felt the only way to get his love was to impress him. Led by her warriors' energy, she went to college and eventually received an advanced degree. When Charlene got married, she did not have or take the time to perform needed household chores. She has not had children. She continues to be driven professionally and this drive has taken a toll on her marriage. Her husband, though professional himself, is not as driven and seeks a more intimate relationship. But Charlene feels confused and overwhelmed by the pressure from her husband. "I've tried so hard. He should be proud of me, impressed by me. My father finally seems impressed with me. He has even come to me for advice. My husband wants more."

Bob, a middle-aged man, was admitted to the psychiatric unit of a hospital because of depression. I saw Bob, his wife, and his 15- and 17-year-old sons in a family therapy session. Each had a story to tell and was eager to tell it. They began with Robbie, the 17-year-old. "Dad gets upset with stupid things. He yells and screams when I don't put tools back where they belong. He has the whole wall of his shop marked with white silhouettes of all his tools where each tool is to be hung. He goes crazy when he finds a tool missing."

Rod was eager to jump in. "Dad is a fanatic about how the lawn is mowed. The last time I mowed it he went crazy because the lines made by the mower were not straight. He should have been happy I did it."

Rhoda, in tears, finally had a chance to speak. Between sobs she attempted to explain how her husband was overly demanding and a tyrant with the boys and her.

For once all the family was speaking up about how they felt about dad. They somehow felt safe with dad down and vulnerable and with a mediator present. His strength to fight back was not there. He had given up.

When Bob finally spoke, he told of how his father was an alcoholic, was never at home or "there" for him, and did not provide adequately financially for the family because all his money went for booze. The family lived in poverty in a dilapidated house. Bob was committed to being different. "I want to be proud of my family and my home. I want my family to be proud of me and how I provide for them. Then I heard my younger son talking on the phone to one of his friends, saying he did not want his friend to come over because his father might be on a rampage. I realized I was a total failure as a father. My son was embarrassed by me. I was embarrassed by the house I lived in when I was his age. I was embarrassed by my father and he is embarrassed by me. In spite of everything I have done for him, for all of them, they are embarrassed." His warrior energy had been directed to being what he felt was a responsible provider, father, and husband. He was a good warrior, a too good warrior.

The warrior energy is not always channeled in a constructive positive direction. This same energy can lead to negative, destructive, criminal behavior.

A 36-year-old man came to therapy because his marriage was in jeopardy. Aaron was the son of a straight-laced minister. Aaron's wife had discovered he was in an extramarital affair, and he came to therapy admitting he had a sex addiction problem. Though his wife was aware of only one affair, there had been many. He was beginning to realize his problem was destroying his life. "As hard as I try to stop (having affairs), and I've tried many times even before Sandy found out, it is impossible for me to stop." Sometimes this warrior energy can be considered an obsession. Aaron was obsessed by sex.

"My father would preach about the evils of all kinds of sex. He would preach about the evils of adultery. He was always preaching, in the pulpit and at home. Whenever he was talking, he was preaching. He never would listen to me. I hated him. When I was sent away to a Christian college, I was a good student, but I would go into the coffee shop and meet people from the other college in town. Soon I had friends from the other college and met some women there. I started having sex. I felt guilty, but it was exciting. I guess it was my way of rebelling. Maybe that is what I am still doing, rebelling against the church, rebelling against my marriage. Even though my dad married us, I have not been to church since college." Sex was Aaron's way to rise above his father in strength. He had found power and strength, though a false power and strength, in his "conquest" of women. His warrior energy was directed to this conquest.

A 16-year-old boy was brought to me by his mother. His parents had been divorced and his mother had to work, leaving little time for Chuck. His father was an impressive professional individual who occasionally took Chuck to the city for major league sporting events. Lacking his father's attention, Chuck found a way to gain fame among his school friends. They were impressed when he told them about and showed them his new possessions, items stolen the night before in his round of burglaries. In his pursuit of fame, he exacted tribute on the community. Since the time I saw him, he spent time in a juvenile detention center and has now served several years in prison. Although his family appeared to be good, loving, and concerned as a family, he felt he had to use his warrior energy to impress his friends to make up for his lack of loving parental attention.

One young woman, Erin, was in her third year of college, taking an excess load of courses and getting straight "A's." While in high school her activities took her to district and state contests where she always did well. She was involved in many extracurricular activities and continued to be very involved in extracurricular activities in college until her "breakdown." In seeing this family in family therapy, one phrase was heard repeatedly from her father: "yes, but. . . ." Whenever his daughter described one of her accomplishments, he would answer "yes, but other things are more important" or "that's nice, but you need to learn to slow down." He had not offered her direct and unconditional acceptance but always included another challenge to her. She was unable to please him. She pushed and pushed herself to get praise she would never get. All her success led to an emotional collapse.

People use many different defenses to deal with the pain of their original trauma. These defenses move the individual toward more and more complete dissociation from the original trauma. For the dissociation to be complete, the individual needs to go beyond this third stage of his or her drivenness to find apparent success to the stage of finding satisfaction in becoming established in family, home, and work. As this warrior energy grows in strength, as goals are reached, the individual reaches beyond to the fourth generation to consolidate his or her energy to become established.

THE FOURTH GENERATION: BECOMING ESTABLISHED

Healfdene prospers with four children. The second, Hrothgar, becomes the fourth King of Denmark and the King of our story. Such are Hrothgar's fame and strength that his kinsmen are eager to serve him as retainers. The number of his retainers increases to become a formidable army. In planting the roots of his kingdom, Hrothgar erects the greatest of banquet halls ever known, Heorot. In this hall he holds feasts and distributes his wealth. In this hall Hrothgar feels secure and free, free as the deer after which the hall is named.

Finally, real success is at hand: the culmination of this lineage of kings, beginning from a castaway and growing in success to the famous, powerful, and established King Hrothgar.

After our hard work to achieve a position in life, after we graduate from college, after we get married or build a home, after our children are born or are up and out, after we retire, after any number of turning points in our life, we finally reach a stage of feeling as if we "have it made." We have become established. We feel safe and satisfied in what we have accomplished. The trauma of our distant past has long been forgotten and overcome. At least, that is what we think. A good portion of the clients in my practice hold this belief of "I've got it made," yet they experience some need to enter therapy.

Cindy, 31 years old, had been married for five years. She had a job she loved, could find no fault with her husband, had her dream home in the country and horses. She "had it made." She knew her friends envied her, yet she became obsessed with a man she had met through her work. This obsession interfered with her love for her husband. He knew something was wrong but knew nothing of her troubles. Cindy believed she was on a path of self-destruction and felt extremely guilty. She knew she could lose her envied life, but she believed she could not help herself.

Johanna, a 60-year-old woman, also had everything she could want. Her husband had done well financially in life and had recently retired. She was looking forward to spending more time with him. He had always seemed so busy, and now he would have time for her. She came to therapy when her husband announced he wanted to leave. To him, Johanna had many problems, was unhappy and complained too much. He did not want to spend the rest of his life in misery. She was about to lose her dream.

A 50-year-old physician came to therapy because of panic attacks. Jacob was controlling the attacks with medication well enough to continue his medical practice. But he knew something else was wrong. His practice flourished. He was happily married. He was very proud of his two children, who were away at college. His wife was excited by her full and beautiful life. Jacob could not understand why he should feel panic.

My practice of psychology is in a rural setting. Raymond had moved to this idyllic setting two years earlier when he was promoted to plant manager in a large manufacturing firm. He and his wife were excited by this promotion and the possibility of raising their three children, ages four to ten years, in this healthy environment. His life seemed perfect, but he found himself becoming irritable and explosive at work and at home. His wife was aware of this personality change and became increasingly concerned.

In each case, the individual reached a stage of success in life, was ready to settle down, and was looking forward to enjoying this established stage. Each was unable to understand the cause of his or her dis-ease. The connection with the trauma early in their life was not apparent to them. After their hard work to reach this fourth stage/generation in their life, the stage of being "established," they were unnerved by the entry of a monster.

22 / GRENDEL AND HIS MOTHER

Returning to the words of Alice Miller (1981), "In everything they undertake they do well and often excellently; they are admired and envied; they are successful whenever they care to be—but all to no avail. Behind all this lurks depression, the feeling of emptiness and self-alienation and a sense that their life has no meaning. They get the feeling they failed to live up to some ideal image and measure they feel they must adhere to." Though one succeeds in dissociating from the original trauma, finds success, and becomes established in life, feelings of emptiness continue to lurk in the unconscious mind.

Hrothgar consolidates all he has gained through the growth of the Danes by building the largest and greatest hall ever known. This hall, called Heorot, the swift hart, becomes famous and supports everyone whom "God has entrusted to" Hrothgar. Now, the benevolent and powerful king within us rules and is strong and free. What more could we want? We now have everything. What is left for this King within us to do? He supports everyone in his kingdom and celebrates his success. We have it all. Do we finally feel loved? Everyone with whom we have contact loves us. Is that enough to prove to us we are lovable? It is very lonely here at the top. We hold no trust that real love exists. Since we were abandoned and not loved, how can we trust others to really love us? Perhaps they love us only because of what we can give them. Even within the security of Heorot, as a deer knows, danger still lurks. Where do we go now?

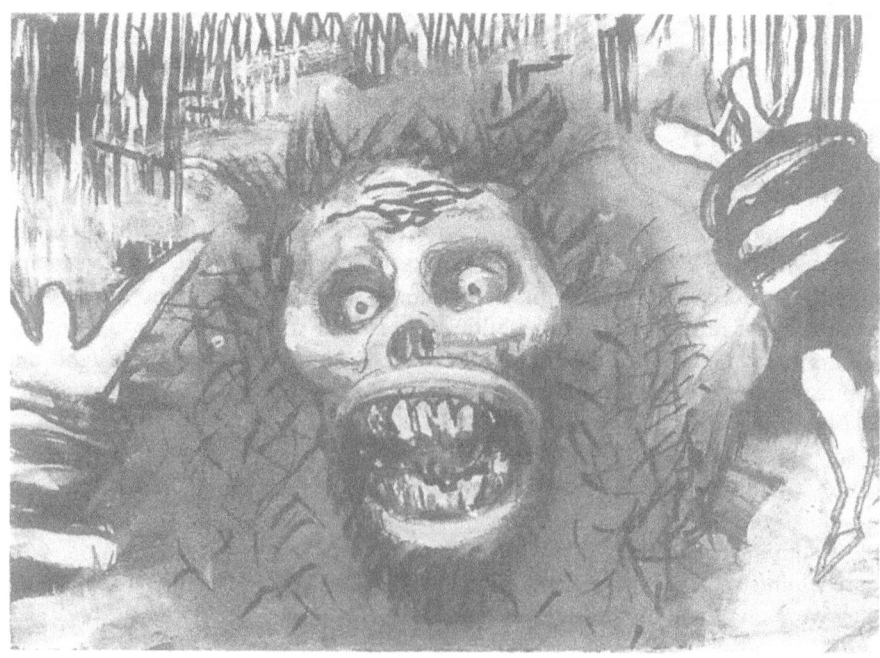

CHAPTER III

Grendel, Our Despair

Hrothgar reaches his pinnacle of strength. His army is formidable with kinsmen ready to serve. He builds the largest banquet hall ever known from which to distribute to his retainers that which God entrusted to him. And he keeps his promise to God at great feasts where he apportions his treasures.

Outside this hall, in the darkness, the monster Grendel stalks. We will soon discover how this fiend has wreaked havoc on Hrothgar's kingdom for twelve years. But first, who is this monster within us? Grendel is something within us that haunts us, causes us emotional and physical pain, interferes with our ability to function at home, at work and at play, and destroys our relationships with others. He is our addictions, our depression, our anxiety. He is our despair.

In this ancient poem Grendel is described in three ways. First he is described as a fiend who wanders the moors and fens of the borderlands, lives in darkness, and suffers greatly. Second, Grendel is a descendant of Cain. His life and unhappiness are attributed to the damnation of God just as God had damned and exiled Cain for having killed his brother, Abel. And third, this fiend from hell is greatly angered and envious of the festivity and joy coming from Heorot, the great hall, joy praising the beauty of God's creation.

GRENDEL OF THE BORDERLANDS

Just as Cain was rejected by God, the Hrothgar lineage began with rejection and abandonment. The pain, though ignored for three generations, still simmers within. We unconsciously ask, "How can I be worthy of such power, wealth, and love, when I was originally not loved but abandoned?" The signs and sightings of Grendel stalking in the borderlands is our feeling of apprehension, a feeling at the edge of our awareness, an undefined feeling of being unloved, a feeling which has its origin in our having been abandoned. "It's not fair, I appear to be loved yet I do not feel loved." We who were abandoned do not trust love because, at a deeper level, we believe that to show love to others is no more than manipulation to gain love. We give in order to be appreciated, but we know as soon as we stop giving, our friends will be gone. We do not trust the love of others, just as we are unable to trust the love of our parents. These beliefs are deep within us and consciously forgotten. These unconscious beliefs are the source of our present problems, causing us emotional and physical pain, bringing us to therapy. Although these beliefs are unconscious, we often experience a sense of apprehension, a sense that something we do not understand is wrong. We know there is something stalking in the borderlands and we are not ready to face it. What is conscious is our success and triumph in the power, fame, and apparent love we have attained.

As these feelings of apprehension grow, Grendel is coming toward Heorot. He eventually enters Heorot in a rage to kill 30 men, to kill part of us at a time when all seems well, to cause 12 years of torment. We do not understand the cause of our despair. But it is this despair that brings us to therapy, that brings us to search for a solution to our problem.

Even though we are not prepared for Grendel to enter, we know he is stomping around the borderlands, the moors, and fens. The borderlands are far away and the most comforting or safest place to keep him. The Grendel within us matches the gloomy damp atmosphere of the moors and fens. We know he would not be happy in the light and noise of Heorot. He would not fit in and he does not belong. We push him out of the way to these borderlands where he is easily ignored. We are dissociated from him, and we are shocked when he finally sneaks into the civilized world of Heorot. Why now? Only because we now feel strong and our strength has prepared us to face him.

Often, clients with symptoms of generalized anxiety speak of a feeling of apprehension, a sense of impending doom. Marlin, a successful attorney, began waking in the morning with a feeling that something bad was going to happen. Why, after all these successful years, did he feel this apprehension? Eventually, after some time in therapy, he recalled one of his favorite high school teachers, saying, "Everyone needs to expect some misfortune in life, life cannot be perfect or totally smooth." Yet, his life had been smooth. He realized that he was unconsciously waiting for something to go wrong and he figured it was about time.

GRENDEL, THE DESCENDANT OF CAIN

Consider Grendel's lineage in the biblical story of Cain:

Genesis 4:1-17 Now Adam knew Eve his wife, and she conceived and bore Cain, saying, "I have gotten a man with the help of the Lord." And again, she bore his brother Abel. Now Abel was a keeper of sheep, and Cain a tiller of the ground. In the course of time Cain brought to the Lord an offering of the fruit of the ground, and Abel brought of the firstlings of his flock and of their fat portions. And the Lord had regard for Abel and his offering, but for Cain and his offering he had no regard. So Cain was very angry, and his countenance fell. The Lord said to Cain, "Why are you angry, and why has your countenance fallen? If you do well, will you not be accepted? And if you do not do well, sin is crouching at the door; its desire is for you, but you must master it."

Cain said to Abel his brother, "Let us go out to the field." And when they were in the field, Cain rose up against his brother Abel and killed him. Then the Lord said to Cain, "Where is Abel your brother?" He said, "I do not know; am I my brother's keeper?" And the Lord said, "What have you done? The voice of your brother's blood is crying to me from the ground. And now you are cursed from the ground which has opened its mouth to receive your brother's blood from your hand. When you till the ground, it shall no longer yield to you its strength; you shall be a fugitive and a wanderer on the earth." Cain said to the Lord, "My punishment is greater than I can bear. Behold, thou hast driven me this day away from the ground; and from thy face I shall be hidden; and I shall be a fugitive and a wanderer on the earth, and whoever finds me will slay me." Then the Lord said to him, "Not so! If any one slays Cain, vengeance shall be taken on him sevenfold." And the Lord put a mark on Cain, lest any who came upon him should kill him. Then Cain went away from the presence of the Lord, and dwelt in the land of Nod, east of Eden.

Grendel, like Cain, is the fugitive who wanders the earth. Cain is damned by God for blaming and killing his brother for his own inadequacies. Grendel is blamed and damned for killing the men of Hrothgar. The Grendel within me blames and kills a part of me, torments me. Grendel continues to carry the burden of his ancestry just as Hrothgar carries the burden of his ancestry, and we carry the burden of our ancestry.

Jamie works as a receptionist and clerk-typist. Because of the economy, several other employees have been laid off and her work load has drastically increased. She is a perfectionist and feels very stressed. She has become very tearful and irritable at work, feeling overwhelmed by everything. Guilt plays a big part in her problem. She cannot say "no" when she needs to. She is feeling more and more inadequate in her job.

In pursuing these feelings, Jamie describes an older sister as assertive and demanding, getting what she wants. Yet, Jamie is afraid to be assertive. She is "damned" to being weak. Why can't she have the strength of her sister. In going deeper, she remembers speaking up to her mother, who, in anger, tells her "you are being just like your sister and I can't stand it." Jamie vows to not be like her sister, and seeks to please by being the perfectionist. She continues to envy her sister's strength, but feels in a bind because this strength upsets her mother. She is "damned" by her envy.

THE GRENDEL OF ENVY

The Lord did not show satisfaction with Cain's sacrifice because, as Cain believed, it did not match up to Abel's offering. The intent of this biblical teaching is that each of us needs to offer our best. When the Lord ignored Cain's offering, Cain felt humiliated, blamed his brother and killed him. Grendel similarly blamed his unhappiness on the joy and happiness heard from the great hall. Blaming his unhappiness on their happiness and festivity, he kills 30 of Hrothgar's men. One way to deal with our torment is to blame others.

The trauma in the childhood of one man, Paul, can best be characterized by the imagery scenario of him as a toddler pulling himself up on the coffee table to explore his environment. He works himself around the edge of the table and is reaching for some object on the table to experience it when the arm of his mother protectively swoops down and grabs him away from the table. He is punished for his curiosity and exploration. He is frightened by the unexpected arm and cries. He is yelled at and put in his crib. If this young child would have had the words to understand what had happened he might have said, "Mom! I need to be handled gently, I need to explore and learn about my environment, my curiosity needs to be supported, I need to be loved and valued." But, those words were not there. All he felt was terror, frustration, and anger. He was incapable of understanding his mother's motives; he only knew that she scared and thwarted him.

Luckily for him, Paul did not loose his need to be curious. His interest in learning continued, and he eventually earned a graduate degree. The trauma of his childhood was lost in the past, and he moved forward to apparent success. What brought him to therapy was a series of failures. He has held a series of jobs, and in each job he began with enthusiasm and moved toward success. But as he moved closer to success, problems began to develop. He became critical of other staff from whom he needed support. He felt they were undermining him. They inhibited his completion of the project. Their arms swooped down to grab him away. His progress toward his goal slowed; more and more fear set in, fear that he would not reach his goal. As he carried a greater and greater burden of fear, his progress came to a halt. He blamed others for his failure. The problems at work increased until he quit or was fired. Grendel stalked in Paul's life: whenever he began to feel success, Grendel came in to destroy it, blaming others for his unhappiness.

When Paul came to therapy, he did not attribute his inability to succeed to early childhood fears and limitations. He blamed his failures on the incompetency and corruption of those who were supposed to support him in his work. It was everyone else's fault. This man was very creative and had high integrity. He could not stand the incompetency and corruption he saw around him. This environment weighed him down, became his Grendel. If we could only kill Grendel, we think, then we could reach our goal of success and feeling loved.

Though she could find nothing greatly wrong with her marriage, 31-year-old Cindy came to therapy because she was having an extra-marital affair, her Grendel. She worked with this man and found him very exciting. As the affair developed, she became more and more critical of her husband, finding fault with him wherever she could. By finding fault, by blaming him, she could justify the affair to herself. On the other hand, she was quick to question whether or not she would be happy if she were to leave her husband for this other man. When Cindy became honest with herself, she realized she was not ready to make a commitment to any man. No matter the relationship, she would want to leave the door open for other men. What was Cindy looking for in men? As therapy progressed, long-term pain was uncovered, the emotional pain caused by her father's lack of trust and respect. He was overprotective and attempted to squash her relationships with any man. She felt unloved by him. As a result, she sought love, trust, and respect from others.

Though she was quick to blame her husband's faults for her affair, Cindy later realized that her affair was an attempt to fulfill her own needs, and thus she could blame only herself. Yet, beyond her own blame, by uncovering the source of her needs, she then could blame her father. Blame is a very complex issue. Cain's tendency to blame his brother is implied in the biblical story, but the real lesson of the story is the lesson of the need to examine our own blame and to take responsibility for our own acts. Something that happened in Cain's early life could have caused him to blame his brother. But what is important is not to blame the historic situation but to use it to understand and eventually transcend our personal needs in the present.

THE GRENDEL OF SELF-BLAME

Another even more common result of childhood trauma is self-blame. How did I bring on this trauma? What did I do wrong? Paul, whose mother swooped him away from the coffee table, described his brother as a placater, always trying to please, a brother who had accomplished nothing important in life. If he had had the words, this brother, when grabbed away from the coffee table, would probably have said, "I'm sorry for what I did, it was wrong of me to try to touch that, I am a bad boy!" With his need to please others, he was frozen in fear, unable to do anything in life.

So many abused women have a need to please others. The woman driven to success to find acceptance from her critical and overprotective father blames herself when criticized. "If I can be perfect, then dad will love me." The sexually abused woman most commonly blames herself. Young girls are commonly taught they need to take care of men, they need to serve them. They feel unable to say "no" to a sexual act or may feel too weak to fight back. Later, they feel guilty for not preventing the abuse from happening.

Traci was in a traffic accident where it was clearly the other person's fault, yet she blamed herself: "If only I had not been in such a hurry to leave work, if I had stopped to talk with the one person who wanted to talk, I would have been a few minutes later and the accident would not have happened. It is my fault." In this woman's childhood, a phrase frequently heard from her mother was "don't rock the boat." Traci was not allowed to express herself and believed it was wrong to do so because expressing herself would upset the peace of the household. She learned early to blame herself if the peace was upset.

Men blame themselves in another way. "I need to provide my wife with everything. When she comes home from work upset about something that happened, I need to provide her with useful advice. I need to be able to solve her problems." With this advice, the wife feels even more irritated or upset because her husband is not being understanding but critical and nagging by telling her what to do. "He does not trust me to know what I should do," she laments. When she shows this irritation, the husband feels even more like a failure because he cannot make her happy. He believes her happiness depends upon him and, when she is unhappy, he blames himself. He then feels unloved because he thinks, "If I cannot make my wife happy, I am not filling my responsibility, and she will not love me. Her irritation proves she does not love me."

With self-blame the blame is internalized. Self-blaming individuals cry, feel remorse, or develop psychosomatic symptoms. However, sometimes a husband who feels guilty explodes and becomes abusive. He is unable to fill his wife's every need, feels guilty, and blames her for making him feel guilty. As in the case of Cain, who blamed others for his feelings of guilt, guilt can lead to abuse. Though Grendel's and Cain's rage was directed at others, the rage had its origin in their own feelings of guilt. Hrothgar, on the other hand, in his feelings of despair over his inability to protect his people, directed his guilt inward in the form of a self-punishing Grendel.

GOD AND ABUSE

Some people believe bad things will happen and always expect the worst: "The world is an evil place and if something can go wrong, it will." Some people with this attitude may believe, "There is no loving God. If there were a loving God, this could not have happened to me." These people may believe in a vengeful God or a God of wrath, or they may deny God's existence altogether. On the other hand, those who continue to believe in a loving God may blame themselves for bringing on abuse. Norah Sargent (Sgroi, 1989) reviews the sexually abuseds' image of God. "How could God let this happen to me?" they ask. The answer is either "I am bad, God is punishing me" or "God is an unfair, vengeful God." A third, more positive alternative might be "God has a purpose for this to happen to me, and, in some way, I will learn or grow from it." Or, "God may not control everything that happens, but God can help me get through it, learn from it and become stronger in the process." Addressing the issue of a client's struggle with and image of God can be useful in the course of therapy (Brink, 1991).

I have found it useful to sometimes ask the question of a client, "What does God look like?" The answers have been very revealing. One woman saw God as a "man in a white robe standing in the sky and looking down on the earth. He does not see me but is looking past me." Mabel considered herself a good Christian but did not feel a "personal relationship with God." In further exploring these feelings, she recalled "my parents would tell me how good my sisters were but never told me I was good." She believed her parents loved her siblings more than they loved her. In the course of therapy Mabel had the occasion to mention this to one of her sisters who then told her she had the same experience. She had never heard from her parents that she was good but she was always hearing how great her sister, my client, was. These sisters felt unloved, though they knew at another level they were loved. If they did not feel their parent's love, how could they expect to feel God's love?

Mike, who claimed to be an atheist, was asked to describe the God others believed in. He described an angry vengeful God. Ralph, who had been born with a physical disability, described a God who did things for him but did not take the time to understand him or his needs. Again, this image of God reflected Ralph's parents' attitude and actions. His parents consistently cared for him, met his needs because of his disability, but they did not take the time to understand how he felt, nor did they realize his need for greater independence.

ATTACKED WHILE ASLEEP

Returning to the poem of Beowulf, late in the evening the celebration and gift giving ends and Hrothgar's men fall asleep in the great hall. Grendel then enters the great hall and savagely slaughters 30 men, carrying them back to his lair.

We are attacked by our tormentor when we least expect it. We would least expect the monster to arrive during the time in our lives when we have become established, feel secure, and are celebrating our success. Yet, the Grendel within arrives and kills 30 of our warriors, robs us of our strength, leaving us feeling even more vulnerable.

Jim, a 42-year-old skilled factory worker, drove to his son's high school in the evening to pick him up from football practice. Jim arrived at the school in a state of panic and just sat in the car, believing he was having a heart attack. As the boys came out of the locker room, one called back to Jim's son, who came running. Seeing the state of his father, the son drove him straight to the emergency room of the hospital. There, he was diagnosed as having a panic attack.

Jim's fear to drive and even to leave the house rapidly escalated. He would break into a sweat if he needed to go somewhere. He did not have a panic attack as severe as the first one for about a month, but then he decided to come for therapy.

Jim prided himself on being a good father, better than his own father who had been abusive when he was at home. When not at home, his father was usually at a bar. Jim prided himself on being there for his son, but when we uncovered the deeper message of his tormentor (his panics), he realized that when he was with his son, he felt awkward and did not know what to talk about. Jim's father never carried on a normal conversation with Jim but was always angry or challenging. Jim was different. He would talk to his son, telling him about his day, wanting to impress his son, wanting his son to respect him, but, behaving as a normal teenager, his son seemed impatient and did not seem to care about his father's daily activities. Jim felt very uncomfortable when alone with his son. While talking about these feelings he could feel himself getting hot and going into a panic. Jim's Grendel attacked him when he least expected it.

GRIEF

When the sun rose, Hrothgar and the remaining retainers see the blood and destruction in the great hall. When they see the trail of blood leading away into the distances, the Danes begin to wail and sing their mourning songs. Hrothgar is lost in grief, unable to act with his heavy heart. Hrothgar fears this monster; fears his lack of power in this situation; feels guilty for being unable to protect his people; and worries obsessively, a worry that grows over the next 12 years of suffering.

Jim was unable to drive himself to the hospital. His panic attack left him totally helpless. This helplessness had these three components: fear, guilt, and obsessive worry. When we consider each of these three tormentors, we better understand the strength of Grendel. Jim feared disappointing his son, felt guilty for not being strong for his son, and obsessively worried about the consequences of his weakness.

Tina, a 30-year-old executive secretary, recently lost her job because of economic cutbacks and low seniority. She had a great need to be strong, to be able to take care of herself in all situations. Though she saw her husband as a strong and competent person, she had made most of the family's major decisions. She selected the house they were buying and the cars they had bought, and she decided when to begin their family. Tina and her husband had an 18-month-old daughter, and she felt good about balancing her job with being a mother. Losing this job triggered a feeling of inadequacy. Tina felt devastated, humiliated at the thought of being "only a housewife." Financially, there was no great urgency to find another job, but Tina realized that no one would want to hire a high-priced executive secretary. She would have to start again at the bottom. She was frightened.

Facing her Grendel, Tina realized she felt like an impostor in her job. She was proud, worked hard, and received many compliments, but she believed she had this job just because of luck, and eventually her incompetency would be found out. She knew the cutbacks were necessary, and it was logical that she be the one laid off because of her low seniority and the nature of her work load. Yet on another level the layoff confirmed Tina's fears of incompetency. The feelings of grief: guilt over working beyond her level of competence, fear of becoming dependent, and obsessive worry were all present. Tina felt severely depressed.

In the course of Tina's therapy, on a rational level she realized that she was competent in her job and that her feeling of being an imposter was irrational. Then she recalled words she heard from her parents as a child: "where were you when the brains were passed out?" "You dummy." At the time, these words had seemed funny but she now knows part of her believed them. Over the years in between she took them as a challenge and wanted to prove to her parents that they were wrong. Tina's depression became anger. She began to feel ripped off by her parents.

Jim's feelings of helplessness and Tina's fear and feelings of failure are examples of King Hrothgar's grief.

FURTHER ATTACKS

After the first night and the murder of 30 men, Grendel returns night after night. In his revenge, in his hate for Hrothgar's success and for God's damnation, and because of his first night's success in the great banquet hall, he is eager to return. He has a taste for blood and wants more.

Once the gates open, the feelings rush in. Once someone has a panic attack, they quickly begin to fear future panics. This fear of fear rapidly escalates as do addictions, extra-marital affairs, and all emotional and behavioral disorders. New behavioral patterns become established, self-supporting and resistant to change. The person who tries to contain rage feels worthless once the rage has rushed forward, making it all the easier for the rage to rush forward again and again. Once a person withdraws in fear of something, the fear grows and the withdrawal escalates. Once a power struggle develops, the feelings of frustration and rage escalate, and the weapons of the struggle seem impossible to put down.

For Tina, being laid off was a beginning, and her feelings of inadequacy rapidly escalated, her Grendel returning night after night. For George, a 48-year-old factory worker, his tormentor was an injured back, a work-related accident. His orthopedist felt surgery was not necessary and ordered physical therapy, indicating that George would become "as good as new." As the time went on, however, his pain continued. The soft tissue damage did not heal as quickly as George had expected, and his physician had not told him that such injuries can take a long time to heal. He was off work and on Workers' Compensation.

After a few months the insurance company requested another evaluation and the physician indicated that George could go back to work, but George knew he could not. He experienced continued pain in his lower back which kept him awake at night or allowed him only a couple of hours' sleep. George knew he could not perform his job. His frustration and anger with his physician, employer, and insurance company grew. This increased frustration and anger increased his pain (Brink, 1989).

Physical tension increases pain. Also, attention to the pain increases the sense of pain. In George's case, each letter, each phone call, each sleepless night caused greater attention to be focused on the pain, intensifying the pain. Such pain is not malingering but real. George's fear, guilt, and obsessive worry played important roles in intensifying the pain; Grendel returned night after night. The fear of failure, the fear he would never be physically whole, the guilt of his inability to support his family and of not living up to his image of a man, and the obsessive worry over these unresolved issues greatly intensified the pain. George's power struggle with his employer and insurance company continued to grow. He was unable to lay down his weapons in this war: his retaining of a lawyer, his letter writing, and, most of all, the pain itself. In this situation, George needed to maintain the pain to justify the struggle, real pain intensified by stress and the focus of attention on the injury. Just as he was unable to lay down his weapons, the insurance company and employer were unwilling to lay down their weapons.

This power struggle was not just external to George, between him and his insurance company and employer. It was also internal, between his disabled, painful self, and his image of himself as a hard-working man who wanted to be healed and return to work, a man of integrity who did anything his employer requested and was always reliable. This internal battle disallowed him from letting go of the physical tension, tension that intensified the pain. Grendel returned night after night, the war and pain continued to escalate, and so did frustration and depression.

WITHDRAWAL TO OUTLYING BUILDINGS

George withdrew more and more. In his depression and escalating pain, he no longer saw his friends. He became more and more self-absorbed. Turning inward in this manner he focused his attention more and more on the pain, intensifying the pain. He was cowering in one of the outlying buildings near the great banquet hall.

After the second night of Grendel's return, Hrothgar and his men begin to realize that the situation is hopeless and find other, safer places to sleep. They know that if they keep out of Grendel's way, they might survive. In the same way, Jim, with his panic attacks, quickly became agoraphobic, fearing to leave the house for fear of having another panic attack. Tina, in her loss of self-confidence, became more and more depressed and her outgoing nature diminished. She stayed home more and more evenings.

Betsy, 26 years old, continued to live with her parents. She worked nights for a cleaning service, generally alone in a suite of doctors' offices. Her employer was pleased with the quality of her work, but she was slower than he would have expected. He paid her by the job and stopped by the offices once or twice a week to check her work. She started at 11 P.M. and, though she had until 8 A.M., when the office staff begin their day, to complete her work, she should have been able to finish the job much earlier, by 2 or 3 A.M. She usually finished by 5 or 6 A.M. While working, when she finished one room, she simply needed to turn off the light and close the door. The last job to do in each room was to wipe off the table, desk, or counter tops. When Betsy got to the end, however, she had difficulty with wiping off the last surface. She did it over and over, saying to herself as she looked around the room, "That's good enough." She seemed to freeze in repetitively wiping off the last surface for maybe five minutes, finally breaking away to stand in the door with her hand on the light switch for an equally long time looking around the room, again saying, "That's good enough." By the time Betsy went through this routine in the dozen or so rooms, two or more hours were added to her work.

Betsy came to therapy because this obsessive-compulsive behavior had gradually gotten worse, taking up more and more of her time. She had the same problem cleaning at home, which greatly irritated her family, especially when they wanted to go somewhere and had to wait for her. This obsessive-compulsive behavior did not seem to interfere with her ability to prepare meals because the family ate in the kitchen, so she did not have to leave. But cleaning up after dinner was a problem.

Betsy's obsessive behavior trapped her in the outlying buildings of the Beowulf story. She never needed to face the world. The textbook cause for obsessive-compulsive behavior is in the payoff it offers as a way to protect oneself from the expression of repressed anger. The structure or ritual of such behavior prevented Betsy from finding herself in a situation where she might lose control. From my experience, this protection from anger seems often to be the case.

Betsy's obsessive behavior brought her to therapy; it was her Grendel. Behind this behavior was her fear of anger, anger at her parents for being overprotective, for not allowing her to date. Though she recently had a date, her parents were once again over-involved, and she believed the man was no longer interested. She was angry.

THE SPIRIT IS BROKEN

Hrothgar and his wife retreat to their chambers. The King feels safe in his chambers, and his closest advisors visit him there with the hope of finding a solution. He maintains his title of King but feels the unkingly feeling of hopelessness. He maintains his belief in God but questions why God is doing this. All he has is his belief in God; otherwise he has given up. All attempts to overcome Grendel have failed.

Fear begets fear. Guilt begets guilt when the situation does not change. Our obsessive worry continues to grow. There appears to be no solution and we talk about "giving up." All our defenses have failed, but we still hang onto them, trying them over and over. We will eventually discover that by truly "giving up," we will find the key, the solution to our problem. But we do not truly give up; we only talk about it, hoping we will be rescued from our pain, hoping for God's intervention. We no longer feel we can solve the problem alone and hope, in our despair, that we will be rescued.

The ultimate expression of the broken spirit is the thought of suicide. Often the threat of suicide is a call for help. Over a period of three weeks I had phone calls from and saw four people: a man who was determined to leave his wife, the wife, her mother, and the couple's adult daughter. The wife was threatening suicide. She and her husband had been married 28 years. They had three children, including two boys, one in the military and the other married and living independently out West. The oldest child, their 28-year-old daughter, continued to live in the area. The wife/mother, Wanda, had been in emotional pain for some time and had been in therapy. Her husband was emotionally detached from everything in his life, and this detachment left Wanda feeling unloved. She begged him for more attention but the more she asked the more he pulled away. "He seems so morose at home but so alive when he is around others," she would say. She could not prove he was having an affair but she expected it. He finally decided he had had enough, and her world collapsed.

Building up to this climax, the pattern of fear, guilt, and obsessive worry was most evident. With her nagging, Wanda attempted to pull her husband closer, but she knew she was pushing him away. She knew it was ineffective, but knew of no other way, feeling afraid, guilty, and worried about what would happen. So, the thing she feared most happened. Her nagging destroyed their life together, and all she could hope was that her talk of suicide would bring them back together. Her spirit was broken and she felt she had to grovel for help.

THE TREASURE-THRONE IS SAFE

Though Grendel enters the great hall every night, he does not go near the throne of Hrothgar. It is blessed by God. The king within us, the blessed throne, the wise and understanding part of us is not destroyed. It is this wise part of us that brings us to therapy.

The unconscious mind strives for health, sometimes in what might be considered bizarre ways. Real change toward health requires we reach "rock bottom." The process of life has its ups and downs, the "downs" coming when we have the emotional strength to survive them. The blessed throne, our wise God within, persists and knows when we are ready to face the tormentors within us.

One exception may be suicide, but many suicides are accidents that occur when a person's threat of suicide is really a cry for help. When our spirit is broken we find ways to call for help from others. Whether or not we consider suicide as a legitimate way to avoid severe emotional and physical pain is an eternal question. For those who believe in an afterlife or reincarnation, suicide may be seen as one stage in further personal growth, or as failure to meet earthly challenges for personal growth with God's guidance. I do not attempt to provide an answer.

Emotional and behavioral problems, when faced, can be recognized as part of the process of striving for greater personal and spiritual health. "Hrothgar's throne" provides us with the continued strength for and faith in this growth.

Gladys, a 68-year-old retired state employee, began therapy because of obsessive worry that her children and grandchildren may be diagnosed as HIV positive. She had a son and two daughters, all married, and she had seven grandchildren, ages six years to 28 years old. All were healthy and had lived life with no severe adversities. Though she felt somewhat estranged from her one son, who seemed to have developed close ties to his in-laws, she did see him occasionally. Though her family was concerned about her obsessive worry, they expressed frustration and impatience with her and attempted to reassure her of their health.

Her worry was an obsessive cry for help, but for what she was not sure. One help in answering her question was the recognition that there was a payoff from her bizarre behavior. Four possible payoffs come to mind. First, one way to express love is to show you care and one way to show you care is by worry. Thus her worry was a way of showing love. A second possible payoff might be that her worry was used for protection. If you worry and think of the worst case scenario, then what happens is bound not to be as bad as expected. The third payoff is related to the second: to worry magically prevents the worst from happening. The fourth payoff is worry as self-punishment for something done wrong in the past, in the present, or for something one might do in the future. If you punish yourself with worry, then God will not need to punish you.

Gladys was living with this fourth payoff. She was punishing herself for what she had done many years before in her indiscretions as an adolescent. She got pregnant and had an abortion. Though she was Catholic and knew the church was against abortion, it did not bother her greatly for many years in her youthful, liberated thinking. But now, since her son was married and showed little interest in his family in favor of his wife's family, she felt she was being punished for her sin. She needed to punish herself to be forgiven by God, and her way of punishing herself was with worry. Her treasure throne, the unconscious God within, offered her a way of penance through the self-punishment of worry, leading her to therapy.

At this stage in the poem, therapy has not begun. Therapeutic interventions and solutions for the many problems people bring to therapy begin in the next chapter. But, in the case of Gladys, the God within led her to psychotherapy to find the answer to her question of why she was punishing herself. With this understanding she found the strength to confess to her family. Her family was supportive. Her confession and her family's support brought her relief from her worry.

PRAYERS TO HEATHEN SHRINES

In the Danes' attempts to find a solution to the problem of Grendel, some advisors suggested praying to heathen shrines. Though Hrothgar maintained his faith in God, we frequently "pray to heathen shrines" in searching for magical solutions to our problems. Gladys's use of worry was a magical way to find relief from her feelings of guilt, her prayer to a heathen shrine, as was Betsy's obsessive-compulsive behavior. Jim's agoraphobia as a way of preventing panic attacks by staying home was a magical prayer to a heathen shrine.

Harvey, a 31 year old, was hospitalized because of his bizarre behavior. As he walked, he would bend over as far as possible. He would exaggerate each step, lifting each foot as high as possible and twisting it upward and inward. His arms would swing wildly to keep his balance in this awkward way of walking. He could only walk short distances because of this exhausting way of walking.

He had always lived with his parents. Though he had worked full time briefly about ten years earlier, he became more and more withdrawn and worked less and less, doing odd jobs, until he stopped working altogether about four years before he was hospitalized. He would spend much time in his room listening to the radio, and when he came out of his room his bizarre manner of walking became more and more extreme.

What was the payoff for this bizarre behavior? The answer came one day when he walked by me at the hospital. I heard him mumbling under his breath, "Watch your step, watch your step." When I watched him walk, I realized he was literally watching each step. This understanding opened a door in therapy. He eventually told me that the phrase "watch your step" was often used by his mother. By being crazy in this manner, by overreacting, by offering this prayer to a heathen shrine, he was punishing his mother for her constant nagging. His manner of walking was his attempt to trample her and free himself from any responsibility.

The prayers to heathen shrines are ineffective solutions to problems. These prayers sometimes work to provide some relief, but they take away from effective or functional living. At other times the prayers cause a great enough disturbance to bring help from somewhere else.

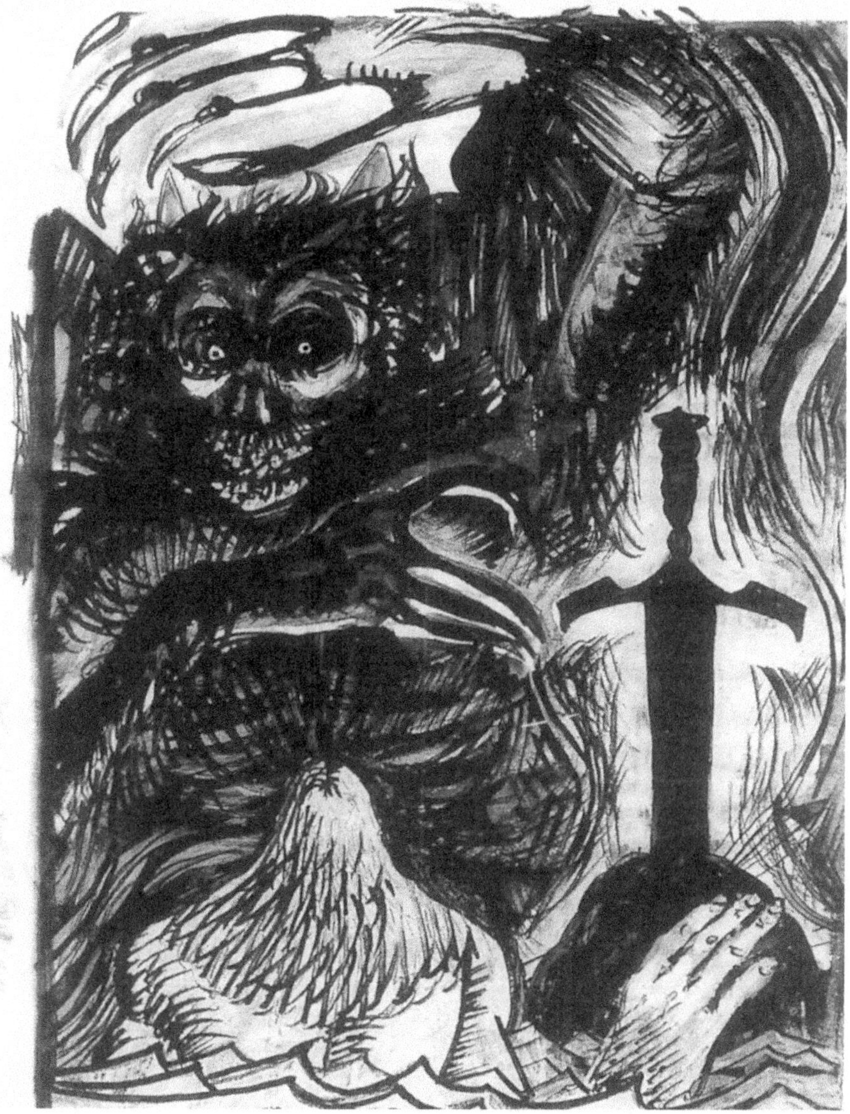

CHAPTER IV

The Coming of Beowulf

Beowulf's arrival begins the quest to resolve Hrothgar's hopelessness, to resolve our deepest torment. Whereas the ancestry of Hrothgar (Chapter II) examines the development of dissociation from our early childhood trauma, and Grendel's attacks (Chapter III) described the nature of the king's and our despair, this chapter begins the quest of the great warrior Beowulf to surmount our torment. This chapter begins the process of therapy, using the techniques of psychotherapy, hypnosis, imagery, and dreamwork to heal the wounds of childhood traumas.

Six clients, Aaron, Craig, Megan, Peggy, Raymond, and Sally, will find resolution of their torment throughout the remaining chapters of this book. Therapists generally see a number of clients each day and need to adjust their frame of reference from client to client, to remember the history and process of therapy of each client from previous sessions of therapy. The reader will need to make similar adjustment in moving from episode to episode of therapy with these six clients.

King Hrothgar had always managed solving problems before. He would assess a problem and then attack it directly, head on. He was invariably the victor. This problem of Grendel is different. None of his weapons or battle strategies work. He has reached the state of hopeless despair. After 12 years of torment he is at rock bottom. He gives up. Before, if he had said, "I give up," giving up was only words. Inside, the power struggle, the war, continued. This time was different. His "human doing" side is no longer effective. A different solution has to be found and it can come only from afar, from across the sea. Hrothgar does not consciously know how to summon this solution, but from deep within the unconscious it is summoned. A young powerful warrior hears the call and sets out to provide Hrothgar with what he needs. Only by giving up conscious control is this solution found.

BEOWULF COMES FROM ACROSS THE SEA

From across the sea, in the Land of the Geats, King Hrothgar's plight is heard in the hall of King Hygelac, the uncle of the great Geat warrior Beowulf. Beowulf, hearing of the plight of Hrothgar, decides to go to the king's rescue. Because Hrothgar had rescued Beowulf's father, Ecgtheow, in his time of need,

Beowulf feels a responsibility, a warriorly duty, to rescue this king. He outfits a ship and selects 14 of the bravest men to take with him. He then leaves for Denmark. After two days at sea these warriors make landfall.

A first step in therapy is to facilitate the warrior within, to lead the client to recognize and call upon his or her inner warrior. The client needs to give up all the other, usual defenses. The warrior within brings the client to therapy—that is, leads the client to do something totally different from the usual, different from the use of his or her usual weapons. It's the warrior within who leads the person to tears when he usually explodes in anger. It's the warrior within who leads the person finally to leave her husband, when she always was the person first to say she was sorry. It is this warrior within who acts bizarrely to gain hospital admission. It is the warrior within who offers new and unique ways to solve a problem. This bizarre or unexpected behavior is not necessarily manipulative but comes from the unconscious mind, from a distant land. The warrior within shows itself when you do something different, something you have never done before, something that brings attention to the problem in a clear and unique way. The bizarre walk of the man "watching his step" was the warrior within taking new steps to find resolution to deal with his mother's nags.

The role of the therapist is to appreciate this cry for help, to confirm for the client that the old ways have not worked and to encourage the client to search, to struggle, and to open oneself to new solutions. The client's pain and struggle are positive signs of health. This struggle is the warrior coming forth, the beginning of the warrior's journey to victory. The client's volunteering to come to therapy is a statement of the client's readiness to use new ideas, new weapons in this struggle to overcome despair. Exceptions to this readiness are clients who involuntarily come to therapy, as ordered by some authority or to appease a spouse or parent.

Recall Raymond, the plant manager who had recently moved to our rural area of Pennsylvania. He came to therapy when his wife expressed a concern or worry for Raymond's change in behavior. He had become short-tempered and irritable with his wife and children. Besides these complaints, he complained of neck and shoulder pain and tension. With his decision to begin therapy, the warrior within began his journey. Therapy had been the last thing on his mind until his wife suggested he needed help. Even then he did not believe help was necessary until the day he blew up with one of his employees. Then he knew. Reassurance that he made the right decision, reassurance that there was an answer within him to explain his new irritability, strengthened his resolve, the warrior within. He became openly curious about why his demeanor had changed. His wife pointed out something to him that, at first, he did not want to believe, but that raised his level of consciousness. He had to admit he was more irritable, not just in his family, but also at work. He did not like this change within him and knew he needed help.

Sally, a lawyer, was sitting across her desk listening to a client complain about his marriage and sex life. His wife was explosive, he said. The littlest things set her off. "I can't even look at her without her exploding." These words brought a rush of feelings to Sally. Her client was describing Sally. She thought she and her husband had a pretty good sex life, but she would go into a rage if her husband would watch her while she was dressing or undressing. She didn't understand this rage and knew it greatly upset her husband. These words from one of her clients convinced her to become a client herself. The warrior within got the message there was a problem and was ready to go to the rescue. Sally knew she needed help.

BEOWULF COMES UNEXPECTEDLY

When Beowulf and his men arrive on the shores of Denmark, neither Hrothgar nor his men expect him. The harbor sentry is surprised to see such a well-armed ship arrive in the daytime: "No armed men have ever ventured to land here so openly," he muses.

We, in our pain, are generally surprised to discover the warrior within when we least expect him. In the time of greatest pain, we find ourselves rising to the occasion, lifting ourselves above the pain. With severe physical pain, the body's natural defense is the release of endorphins and numbness. With emotional pain we find an emotional numbness which can be reinterpreted as a sense of quiet strength. As a hobbyist bee keeper, I recall falling, while collecting a swarm of bees from high up in a tree. The fall that took only seconds seemed like minutes, allowing me enough time to decide on which branches I should grab to break my fall. My unconscious warrior arose in a time of emergency.

Craig worked at the management level for a large factory. He frequently distributed memos and reports to the higher levels of management and directed and served the lower levels. In the process of his daily work he found himself checking and rechecking his work, checking and rechecking the words in his reports, fearing he might include something that would offend someone else at the plant. This process of checking and rechecking caused him to get behind in his work. One of his supervisors said to him one day, "I thought I would get this yesterday. What took you so long?" Craig was proud of his work and very much embarrassed by this comment. He got the message and knew he needed to seek help.

After hearing his story, I made the comment to Craig, "Such obsessive-compulsive behavior is not unusual. In fact, if another therapist mentions a person is a 'checker,' we know what is meant. I have worked with a number of 'checkers' and they have found relief once we get to the cause of the problem. Your fear of offending someone is not unusual. When your fear becomes the obsession that checking is to you, the fear is real and is coming from a part of you that would like to say something offensive or believes it would be too easy to say something offensive. Though you may not be aware of this deeper need to offend, of some deep resentment or anger, we need to explore the possibility, to learn where it comes from."

This comment was reassuring to Craig. This reframing comment gave him a new perspective on his problem, signaling the arrival of the warrior. He felt he had made the right decision to come for therapy. A part of him knew, unconsciously if not consciously, that his checking was a symptom of deeper resentments. Such understanding comes when least expected, often unconsciously before it becomes conscious.

The first personal awareness of the arrival of the warrior within is often facilitated through the reframing of a client's belief by the therapist. The internal beliefs that anxiety or depression are terrible afflictions are reframed to the beliefs that anxiety or depression are messages from the unconscious mind, or from God. These messages need to be faced and understood to be resolved. When reframed in this way, the messages signal the arrival of the warrior, providing the client with reassurance and relief.

Aaron came to therapy because his marriage was in trouble. He had been having one extra-marital affair after another. During the first session he was most afraid of his wife's rejection, especially remorseful and committed to ending the affairs. I suggested to him "if every woman on this earth would tell you they loved you and would make love to you, you still would not feel loved. If just one person rejects you, you believe you are not loved. To really feel love you must first be able to love yourself, you must first believe you are lovable. Your affairs are a message to you, telling you you have a problem, pointing to your feeling of inadequacy, to your belief of being unlovable. We need to resolve this problem."

Aaron's problem was reframed from that of his wife rejecting him to a problem of feeling unlovable. I did not condemn him for his affairs but provided him with some understanding, understanding that made sense to him whether conscious or unconscious. He felt reassured he was on the right track. If he had thought the goal of therapy was to end having affairs and to live a monogamous life, he would have panicked, and a barrier to change would have been built. He would rather have found a way to "have his cake and eat it too," to keep his wife and continue the excitement of having affairs. For Aaron, beginning therapy was a way to appease his wife and not change. He would have had difficulty believing living a monogamous life could be satisfying and fulfilling, but the new goal of learning to love himself seemed safe to him.

As I was working on a report the phone rang. A woman's voice spoke, "I need an appointment." I asked her about the nature of her problem. She complained, "My husband is unhappy. In spite of everything I do, in spite of my hard work and the money I bring home, I just can't make him happy."

I commented, "Your husband wants more of your time for himself and you feel really pressured by it." This jump in logic surprised her and was trance inducing. She was silent for a moment then sighed. The voice continued, but in not such desperation. "When can we see you?" When the appointment was made she identified herself as Megan. Reframing the problem from her husband's unhappiness was an unexpected surprise.

Reframing as a therapeutic technique is found in the literature on hypnosis, though using it does not involve direct trance induction. When an important issue is reframed, it is a startling experience, an experience that catches one's attention, an experience that, in itself, induces a trance or different awareness. The reframing experience comes as a surprise; it comes from afar, from across the sea.

THE SENTRY TRUSTS BEOWULF

The arrival of Beowulf's ship in daylight surprises the Sentry. The Sentry trusts Beowulf when he arrives with such openness. The growing feeling of trust comes with the feeling of surprise, the "ah ha!"—the feelings of relief, curiosity, and insight that arrive when the problem is effectively reframed.

Raymond, 38 years old, moved to rural Pennsylvania to become a plant manager. He was excited about his promotion and believed this rural setting would be a better place to raise his children than in the city. But, he had become irritable and explosive at home and at work and was suffering from neck and shoulder tension. His irritability was noticeable and his wife began to complain. He was a rational man who thought things out in detail before making decisions. His decision to move here seemed very right to him, but, he admitted, something was wrong. "Being this way is ridiculous. At first I refused to believe my wife that I was different, but one day I blew up at a guy at work and it scared me."

Raymond grew up in Philadelphia, met his wife in high school, went to college in the city, earned his B.S. in mechanical engineering, got married, and found a good job in a large factory in the area. He had led an apparently ideal life, was intelligent, and knew his behavior was inappropriate.

During our second session I hooked the Galvanic Skin Response (GSR) biofeedback sensor to his finger. This procedure was a little unusual, but Raymond was an engineer and a rational person. I thought it might interest him to see how his body reacted emotionally to various thoughts.

We continued talking, first about his life in the city. He and his wife had lived near both sets of parents. They were very close to their parents, who were very involved in the lives of their three grandchildren. The family still returned to Philly two and sometimes three weekends a month to visit their parents.

As the conversation continued, I mentioned, "Now, without your parents in your backyard, you have much more responsibility in caring for the children." Raymond's father was an engineer, too, and he enjoyed talking to his father about his work. I also mentioned his increased responsibility as a plant manager and the fact he had no one to whom he could easily run when he had plant problems. With both of these comments that occurred several minutes apart, the GSR reading on the monitor spiked. The big "R-word," responsibility, was apparently the emotional trigger. At first he denied this was an issue, but he could not deny the GSR response. He did not want to admit the reality of his emotional side, but he was forced to realize the power responsibility had in controlling his life.

When he was able to accept the power of this word, he trusted that we were on the right track.

Peggy came to therapy because of her night terrors and panic. Peggy had grown up in a moderate-sized city and received her AA degree to be a paralegal from a business college in that city. She had recently moved to the area after finding her first job. She had an apartment and was enjoying her first experience being on her own. She then met Russ and felt very good about her relationship with him. Though she occasionally woke in the night feeling exhausted and anxious, she had written these episodes off to nightmares or stress. Peggy had had occasional nightmares when living with her mother. She remembered her mother comforting her in the middle of the night when she was younger, but her mother did not seem greatly concerned. Her mother assumed all people occasionally had nightmares and did not attribute them to any specific problem or to living alone.

One night, when her boyfriend stayed over, she woke him screaming. She had never been told she screamed in her sleep, but at least this time she did. He was terrified. But it felt good to Peggy to have him there to hold her, and she was able to fall comfortably back to sleep.

In the morning over a cup of coffee, Russ suggested she see a psychologist about her nightmares. That was a new idea to her. The only such help she had ever received was in high school when her teacher sent her to see the guidance counselor when she had a boyfriend problem and did poorly on a test. She felt indifferent about that experience.

As the weeks passed, Peggy would occasionally complain to Russ about being tired because she did not sleep well and Russ would again suggest she see a psychologist. Russ had seen a psychologist and found the experience helpful to his problem. He thought she should see me. After some thought, Peggy realized her life would be more comfortable if she could sleep better. She made the decision to make an appointment once she got on her firm's medical insurance policy. By the time she saw me, Peggy was looking forward to the time when she could wake feeling rested. She hadn't paid much attention to her fatigue since she was used to it, but now she began to realize she was almost always tense and tired. She believed, "If I could wake up feeling rested, my life would be perfect." She was on her way to the shores of Denmark.

During the first session of Peggy's therapy I suggested that she was on the right path. I mentioned I was impressed with her ability to let go of her anxiety and fall back to sleep when she had a nightmare. I suggested that when she wakes in the middle of the night, she do what she usually does to relax, possibly stretch, check out the room to get her bearings, take a few deep breaths, check the time and say to her self, "great, I have 'x' number of hours to sleep, I will find a relaxing position to snuggle, relax and let myself fall back to sleep." I also explained to her that these nightmares indicated something was bothering her, and it would be our job in therapy to learn what that something is. Though she did not remember her dreams, I suggested, "When you go to bed, ask your dreams to give you a gift of understanding and, when you wake in the night or wake in the morning, lie there a few minutes to check if you can remember what you were dreaming. If you remember something, write it down. Be curious and patient. Don't try too hard. Eventually you will begin to remember your dreams, and they can help provide you with greater understanding." I explained to her the typical sleeping-dreaming pattern for adults (Buchholz, 1988): the first period of dreaming occurs for about 15 minutes during the second hour of sleep, and the second period of dreaming occurs during about the first half of the fourth hour of sleep. After the fourth hour, sleep is very shallow; a person is in and out of dreaming for much of the next three hours. She agreed she usually gets at least four hours of sleep before she wakes with a nightmare. Explaining this sleep pattern to her and showing her the chart helped her understand her sleeping, dreaming, and waking pattern and gave her confidence that her experience of sleep was not unusual.

Peggy found validation in her new knowledge of the normal sleep pattern and felt we were on the right track. Her inner sentry trusted she was on the right journey.

BEOWULF'S WEAPONS ARE LEFT AT THE DOOR

As the story goes, the harbor sentry appoints officers to guard Beowulf's ship and escorts Beowulf and his men part way up the hill to the great hall of Hrothgar. When the warrior and his men arrive at the great hall they arrange their weapons along the palace wall and seat themselves on benches awaiting an audience with King Hrothgar. While waiting, one of Hrothgar's chieftains questions these men about their lineage. Each party in this interchange is careful to avoid threatening the other. Laying their weapons aside and seating themselves were signs of trust. The sentry's cooperativeness facilitates this trust. Now, explaining their lineage is the beginning of friendship.

Whereas, in the past, we confronted our tormentor with all our defenses and willpower, we now lower these defenses to build within ourselves a new sense of trust. The warrior within becomes open and honest in speaking to our other parts within in preparation for an audience with our inner wise but troubled king. We move surely but cautiously toward greater self-confidence and understanding, testing the validity of this understanding each step of the way.

Both Raymond and Peggy had cautiously lowered their defenses, and both had found a new sense of strength and power in being open and honest. Raymond had used two defenses: denial, denying his problem of becoming irritable; and control, controlling his emotional expression. The biofeedback experience of the previous session had forced him to see these weapons in a new light. He was prepared to leave these weapons at the door, though he needed repeated reminders to lay down his defense of emotional control in many therapy sessions. Defenses can be a very ingrained part of an individual. Peggy cautiously accepted the belief she needed help, but the experience of the first session reassured her she was doing the right thing—she laid down her weapons, her denial and cautious nature.

Megan and her husband also came to therapy. Her husband took charge to explain that Megan was depressed, an "empty shell." She took no interest in her husband and seemed to come alive only when she went to work. She admitted work was important to her. Her husband, however, wanted or needed some recognition, needed to feel her love. When asked how she could show him her love, her first thought was that he should be happy and pleased she was helping the family by working. To her, financial support of the family was very important. I could understand how Megan felt pressured, as she mentioned on the telephone, and I could also understand her husband's frustration. My image of Megan in this therapeutic transaction was that also of an empty shell. Her mind was racing, thinking of what she should or could say but with no identity, revealing nothing of herself.

I offered her an hypnotic exercise and she accepted. I began with a trance induction: "Turn your mind inward . . . experience what you are feeling, notice the feeling of the ring on your finger, the feeling of the collar of your blouse against your neck. Notice the feelings of the snugness of your shoes on your feet. Look deeper to other feelings within you . . ." After continuing in this way for several minutes, using the elevator technique I learned from Peter Bloom, I suggested, "In front of you, you see an elevator door. Next to the door is a button with an arrow down. Above is a panel of numbers, numbering from G, for ground, and down, down to one, two, down and down, to ten and down deeper to twenty, to fifty, and down deeper and deeper. Push the button next to the door. The door opens and you step in. You first look around inside the elevator and see a panel of lights above the door. G is lit up. Next to the door is a panel of buttons. You reach out and push a button. The number in the button lights up. Read me the number that is lit." Megan had selected floor seven.

"The elevator door closes and you feel the elevator begin to move down. The G light goes off and the 1 light goes on. As you go down you are curious and wondering, carrying your feelings with you. The 1 light goes off and the 2 light goes on. The 2 light goes off and the 3 light goes on. Your are curious and wondering as you go down. The 5 light goes off and the 6 light goes on. The 6 light goes off and you feel the elevator slowing down and stopping as the 7 light goes on. The door opens and you look outside the door. Tell me what you see as what you see becomes clear to you."

She reported she saw nothing. She became noticeably anxious. But seeing nothing is important and not at all unusual. As reassurance to her that seeing nothing was important, I automatically continued, asking her to "look into the nothingness. What is it like? Is it hot or cold?"

She answered, "Cold!"

"Is it damp or dry?"

Megan indicated "Damp."

"What else can you tell me about the emptiness? Does it have a color?"

Her answer was "Black."

"Now, some people are able to sense the depth, height, and width of this nothingness. What does it feel like to you?"

"It's small, like a closet, like I'm sitting on the floor of a closet."

"Which way are you facing, the front, back or a side of the closet?"

"The back."

"Can you turn around and face the front?"

"Okay."

"Now look down at the bottom of the door. Can you see some light coming in from under the door?"

"Yes."

"Can you feel the warmth of that light?"

"No. It's cold. I can hear them fighting, yelling out there." (I try to avoid "no" as a response because it lessens the depth of trance. My mistake, but I accept her "no" and continue.)

"Okay, listen to the fighting. Feel the anxiety, the emptiness you feel inside. Stay with that feeling. Feel it in your stomach or chest. You may feel it like a tightness in your chest or you may feel somewhat sick to your stomach."

I could see Megan slightly nodding in agreement.

"Now, let your adult self, with all her wisdom and understanding, go back and sit in the closet with your younger self. Put your arm around that younger self. Show her you understand. Love her. You, better than anyone else, knows how your younger self feels."

Megan began showing some resistance and then her eyes opened. She exclaimed she could not do it, her younger self was so pitiful and disgusting. She was embarrassed by the weakness of her younger self. She should know how to handle the fights of her parents. "After all, I want Dad to be proud of me."

"Okay, back up for a minute. Relax, go back to the darkness, go back to sitting in the closet." After giving her time to return I continued, "Feel your fear and anxiety. Feel the coldness outside the closet. Feel the trapped feeling, feel the feeling of wanting your dad to be proud of you, and also feel the fear, anxiety you have of your parents fighting, of your dad fighting. Feel trapped between the feelings of want and fear. Feel the confusion in your younger self. Your adult self knows your younger self could do nothing to stop the fight. Dad may have been proud of you if you could have said the right thing. Your adult self knows there was no right thing your younger self could say. Let your younger self be a child. Your adult self knows children need to trust their parents and feel safe with them. Children cannot be responsible for breaking up fights. Let your younger self be a child, feel the fear and confusion of a child. In that way you can show your younger self love and she can feel free."

With this hypnotic speech, tears came to Megan's eyes. She laid down her weapon, her need to impress her father, her need to control.

We so often try to change things in our life through willpower. Young Megan thought she should have some way to stop her parent's fights. But willpower is just another way to fight, while letting go of the need to control oneself or others is the first step to finding a solution. Megan had learned the importance of control early in her life, and when she let go of the control in this one exercise, she found she was able to accept her fear and confusion and find a sense of relief. She would return many times to her need to control or be in control, but, eventually, she would discover the real power of letting go. Therapy would offer her repeatedly the power of letting go, of leaving her weapons at the door, so letting go could become a new way of life to her.

Aaron, who had had a number of extramarital affairs, was obsessed with sex. His father was a minister who preached the evils of sex. Aaron related a dream during an early session of therapy. An attractive young woman was sitting on a simple plank bench wearing a white tennis outfit. Behind her was a concrete block wall, a setting reminding him of a gym hallway. She was looking at Aaron and saying "All I want to do is love you." He described his feeling when hearing her statement. "The feeling of love was so simple and pure. There was no baggage of responsibility."

Soon after having this dream, Aaron saw the movie "Sleeping with the Enemy" with Julia Roberts. After the character played by Julia escapes from her abusive husband and settles down in a small mid-western town, she falls in love with the guy next door. Julia has started her life over and refuses to reveal her history to anyone. At one point in the movie, the guy next door complains to her that he does not know anything about her and feels frustrated because she will reveal nothing of her past. Aaron's reaction was, "But that would be wonderful, all that history is unnecessary baggage. Wouldn't it be great to fall in love with no such history. The unencumbered love of the woman saying in the dream 'all I want to do is love you' seems so free, so unencumbered. No history, no responsibility, unconditional love."

Aaron's relationship with his wife, in contrast, was so complicated, so burdensome, especially since she had found out about his affairs. She did not trust him, was paranoid and always nagging him about what he was doing with his unaccounted-for time. "Why can't love be free of such burdens?" Aaron felt exhausted in his relationship with his wife. Love with his wife felt conditional, requiring faithfulness.

Aaron realized the power, the carefree feeling of letting go of control, at least when his wife was not nagging. He granted her the right to be upset with him for his affair(s), but he wanted uncontrolled, unconditional love. He could easily lay down his weapon, his need to be in control, but his wife's nagging quickly caused him to pick it up again. This realization of his and her needs made it easier for him to allow her to express her pain without fighting back. He still could not see himself ending all extramarital affairs, because the "unconditional love" of an affair felt so free and great. However, this dream offered him an early understanding of his wife's and his conflicting needs. His increased patience and understanding helped him lower his defenses and his need to control.

HROTHGAR'S CHIEFTAIN TRUSTS BEOWULF

Megan and Aaron were both in the process of letting go of their defenses, their weapons, their need to be in control. When they gave up control, they both felt the sense of relief of letting go of this big burden, the burden of needing to be in control. Letting go of control opened the door for a greater sense of trust in their lives.

Trust begets trust. Each step of the way, from coming ashore, to being greeted with a tentative sense of trust, to laying down their weapons, to meeting Hrothgar's Chieftain with an even greater sense of trust, strengthens the escalating spiral of trust.

Wulfgar, a trusted chieftain of Hrothgar, meets Beowulf and his men at the door of the great hall. This chieftain questions the soldiers about their lineage, and in this way, they become acquainted. Wulfgar then approaches the king with the announcement of the soldiers' arrival and their request for an audience.

Peggy came to therapy because she had been experiencing night terrors and panic. Early in therapy I suggested an hypnotic exercise for relaxation. The acceptance of an hypnotic exercise and the depth of trance requires growing trust, trust of the sentry at the harbor growing to the trust of the King's chieftain. Following is an abridged form of the trance induction used with Peggy with suggestions for reframing the meaning of her panic and forming a therapeutic attitude for facing the panic.

"Sit back and relax. Let your eyes close. Turn your mind inward—examine the sensations of your body. Take some time to examine these sensations. Notice the feeling of the watch on your wrist, the tightness of your jeans across your knees, the warmth between your back and the back of the chair. Notice the deeper feelings of tension and relaxation within you.

"Now, imagine a warm blue glow starting at the base of your spine. Feel the warmth at the base of your spine, and let the warmth begin to spread upwards to your stomach, melting away tension, stress and strain. . . . Let it spread from your stomach up your back, let it spread up into your heart and lungs, your chest, melting away stress and strain. . . . Feel the warm, heavy, tingling sensation of relaxation in your stomach, heart and lungs. Let the warm blue glow spread to your shoulders and neck, melting away any tensions, stress and strain. Feel the warm, heavy, tingling feeling of relaxation spreading to your shoulders and neck. Let it spread over your face, relaxing your mouth, your nose, the sinuses around your nose, your eyes, the sinuses around your eyes, your forehead, spreading to the top of your head. Feel the warm, heavy tingling feeling of relaxation in your face spread to the top of your head. Let it spread down the back of your head, down around your ears, through your ears, down through the center of your head. As the warm blue glow spreads through the center of your head, let it quiet, slow and relax the thoughts in your head. Watch your thoughts come and go. Imagine where they are coming from and going to. As they come and go, let the warm blue glow slow, quiet the words. Let the words fade. Let the warm glow spread down, back through your neck, across your shoulders and into your arms, relaxing your arms, melting away any tension, stress or strain, relaxing your lower arms, and your hands. Feel warm and heavy.

"Now notice those parts of you that are the most relaxed. Notice the relaxation in your arms and shoulders. Notice how heavy your hands are, resting in your lap." The relaxation in her arms and hands was observable. "Feel the warmth between your hands." Her fingers were intertwined. "And between your hands and your lap. Feel the comfort and relaxation of that warmth. Now notice within you the places of greatest tension. Notice any tension in your chest." Peggy was breathing in a labored way from her chest, not her diaphragm. Her chest was rising and falling, not her stomach. "Now focus for a few minutes on your breathing and let it move downward. The natural, relaxed way to breath is to let your stomach rise and fall. As the air fills your lungs, let your lungs push downward on your diaphragm, the membrane separating your lungs from your abdomen. As your diaphragm is pushed downwards, you stomach is pushed out. Now, let your lungs fill with air and feel them pushing downwards, pushing out your abdomen. When you breathe in this way, there is very little movement of your chest. Your ribs across your chest are rigid. Breathing from your chest is harder and heavier. Breath from your abdomen. With each breath, inhale a sense of calmness and, as you exhale, let that calmness flow deeper. Relax deeper and deeper.

"Now, recall for a moment those moments when you experienced the feeling of panic. Take with you the thought that this panic is emotional pain, and, like any pain, is a message that something is wrong. Consider your panic a message from your unconscious mind. Be curious and wondering. When this panic wakes you or you experience it at other times, be curious and wondering. Be patient while waiting for understanding of this message. You will soon gain understanding of this message. When you understand this message you will have some understanding of what you need to do. Be curious, wondering and patient while waiting for this understanding.

"Now take a few more breaths. With each breath relax deeper. When you are ready, in a few moments, your attention will come back to this room and you will open your eyes feeling relaxed and curious."

Peggy was amazed I knew where she was relaxed and where she was tense. Because of this she gained greater trust in herself for making the decision to enter therapy and for the process of therapy and hypnosis, the trust of Hrothgar's chieftain for Beowulf.

By allowing herself to go into trance, Peggy had left behind her old weapon of willpower. She had used willpower in her attempts to control her panic. By leaving behind her old weapons she found greater trust in her life. A part of her, the wise chieftain within, knew she could trust this warrior within, the warrior who was leading her to change. In moving from the trust of the sentry, to the trust of the warrior, and, eventually, the trust of the king, the wise and understanding part of us, our trust of change, grows in intensity and reality.

Sally came to therapy because of sexual problems with her husband of three years. She felt they could have great sex, and they were generally very uninhibited together. But, when she dressed or undressed and saw Bart watching her, she flew out of control in a rage. She didn't understand the source of this anger. Afterwards, she felt terrible and looked for a time when she could initiate sex to make up.

The first session consisted of history taking. Sally denied sexual abuse in her life. Her step-father, Bob, worked hard, provided well, and enjoyed going to a bar a couple of nights a week. She did not feel especially close to him, but on the other hand, she got along okay with him. She has a brother, four years older than she, with whom she fought "like most brothers and sisters." He was married and lived in the area, but she rarely saw him and didn't seem to care that she didn't see him. Her mother was a caring and loving mother whom she saw or talked with on the phone at least three times a week. Though she could become annoyed with her mother when she gave advice, again, "that's the way mothers are." She remembered screaming at her brother and, occasionally, at her mother, but again feels her behavior was not unusual. I asked Sally about her dreams, and she reported she generally did not remember them. I asked her to pay attention to them when she had them.

Sally came to the next session low keyed, but halfway through the session she mentioned she had had a dream. "In my dream I was screaming. I was standing on a chair and lifting my skirt. You won't believe this, but on the floor was a rat in a clown suit, standing on its hind legs looking at me. That's all there was to the dream."

I laughed. "It conjures up an image of a circus skit. I like it. What part of you is standing on the chair screaming and pulling at your skirt?"

"What do you mean?"

"What are your feelings, standing on the chair and pulling at your skirt?"

"Well, I'm scared."

"Go on, take the feeling farther."

"I'm scared of the rat. It's disgusting."

"How do you feel about the clown costume?"

"I guess it should be funny, but I don't see it as funny. It's disgusting."

"Okay, can you identify some aspect of yourself, some way you are that feels scared and disgusted?"

"Yea, I guess when I go into a rage when Bart is looking at me."

"Okay, now, consider the rat. It's wearing a clown costume. Try to experience what is going on inside the rat. What is the rat thinking or experiencing?"

"Well, it's looking at me. It's curious. It must think I'm crazy, screaming and standing on a chair."

"Tell me what it sees."

"It's looking up at me. It sees me standing on the chair, holding up my skirt.... I just had a funny thought, or feeling. I don't think I was wearing anything under my skirt."

"Okay, again, put yourself in the rat. It is wearing a clown costume. What is the rat's feeling?"

"It's clowning around. It shouldn't be looking under my skirt, but he thinks it is okay because he is just joking around."

"Okay, part of you is doing something you shouldn't, but it's okay because you are just joking around. Can you find that part of you?"

"Sometimes, Bart and I like to spend the evening naked. We'll have dinner wearing nothing and after dinner we will eventually have sex. That usually happens after I have had one of my fits, and when he comes home from work, I meet him at the door naked. It's just joking around. In one way, I think it's disgusting or wrong, but it's okay, we're married, it's defiant and it's fun and exciting."

"How does Bart look at you then?"

"It's okay then, he can look at me with his big eyes and he can lick his lips, but he is just clowning around and it's okay. It's funny, I enjoy it."

"Wow! Sometimes it is okay when you're being funny, but when life is serious, when you are getting dressed to look professional when you go to work or are undressing in a more serious way, then his looks are not okay."

"Yeah, isn't that weird?"

The rat in the clown costume will be an important image later in this book. For the moment, this experience generated considerable trust. Sally opened up and admitted some important things. Her openness suggested that she felt my emotional support in the pursuit of understanding and that she learned some things about herself. Several doors were opened, increasing her trust that therapy was progressing in the right direction toward a solution. Hrothgar's chieftain trusted Beowulf.

HROTHGAR KNOWS, TRUSTS, AND APPRECIATES BEOWULF

The next several stanzas of the poem alternate between Hrothgar expressing his appreciation of Beowulf and Beowulf expressing his prowess in fighting. Hrothgar opens his audience with Beowulf by recalling that he knew Beowulf when he was a lad. Beowulf's father had lived with the Danes and was an old friend of Hrothgar. Hrothgar says to Beowulf, "I am sure God sends you to help the Danes in their struggle against the terror of Grendel!" Beowulf is a welcomed visitor, given the gifts of a hero and a place to sit in the court of Hrothgar. The new warrior within finally wins the trust of our inner king, giving us a great new sense of assurance of being on the right journey.

Sally came to the next session with great enthusiasm and trust. The king within her trusted her warrior's journey to resolution. She had become aware of a connected but new dimension. As a professional person, when she saw clients, she could feel the eyes of some men undressing her. Though she was disgusted by them, it was her profession to listen to them carefully and not let her feelings interfere. She always wore professional-looking suits that were minimally seductive. In her professional life, she could ignore those looks. Only in her personal life, her home life, did it bother her. She shouldn't have to protect herself when at home, she thought. She should be able to just be herself. This realization had sunk in during the week and she was excited about it. She has gained trust in her new insight.

Peggy, who was suffering from night terrors and panic, had taken the hypnotic suggestions that her panics were a message from her unconscious mind and that she should face her panics with curiosity and wonder. At the next session she recalled two nights when she woke screaming. She recalled thinking with curiosity and wonder about the experience the next day, wondering about the message. On the morning of this therapy session she woke with some anxiety and lay in bed for a couple of minutes curious and wondering. She dozed off for a moment and had a faint feeling of something bad happening and a sense of dim light. (Her usual routine is to wake up and get ready for work while it is still dark out.) In Peggy's dream her sense of light was daylight but with the shades pulled, an amber dim light. She felt there was a memory somewhere in the back of her mind that wanted out. Peggy's progress indicated her trust in this therapeutic journey—Hrothgar recognizes and trusts the strength of Beowulf.

Returning to Raymond, the logical next step in therapy was to use the word "responsibility" as the affect bridge (Watkins, 1971) in time regression (Barnett, 1981). Trance was induced: "Sit back and relax. Close your eyes and imagine standing at the top of a flight of stairs. It's a long flight with 30 steps. At the bottom you can see a door with a frosted glass window. Notice the light shining through the window shines on the bottom several steps. Count the number of steps in the sunlight. How many are there?" He answered, "Three." "Good. Now you are going to begin walking down the steps as I count them. Thirty, twenty-nine, twenty-eight." I counted following the rate of his breathing. "Twenty-seven, taking one step at a time, relaxing deeper and deeper. Twenty-four, twenty-three, feeling the weight of your body being carried along by your legs, your arms swinging freely, Nineteen, eighteen, a step at a time, relaxing deeper and deeper, fifteen, fourteen, watching the distance between you and the bottom of the stairs becoming shorter and shorter, relaxing deeper and deeper, ten, nine, eight, soon you will be at the bottom, five, four, three, two, one. Now reach out and take hold of the door knob, turn it and push the door open. Take a few steps out into the sunlight into a garden. A few steps from you is a comfortable lounge chair. Take those steps to the chair, sit down, sit back and relax, deeper and deeper."

"As you sit there relaxed, recall the feeling of responsibility. Take the feeling of responsibility with you as you begin to go back through time. Watch your life go by, day by day, week by week, year by year, watch the seasons, holidays, people, places go by, while carrying responsibility with you. As you go back through time, be curious and wondering. Watch your life go by. Soon something will catch your attention; it may surprise you. Be curious and wondering. When something catches your attention raise the index finger of your right hand to let me know—as you go back through time, taking your responsibility with you, being curious and wondering."

Raymond's finger rose.

"Okay, stay where you are in time and tell me what's happening."

"I'm at my old job as an engineer, about five years ago. I am walking into my boss's office curious about what he wants. He has another job for me. I think, 'how am I ever going to get to it,' but I don't say anything."

"Now what happens?"

"I ask him some technical questions about it and leave the office . . ."

"Okay, go back to your work area, sit down at your desk and do what you need to do to express your frustration—maybe rest your head on your arms on your desk, or lean back resting your head on the back of your chair, or wring your hands together. Do what you need to do to express your frustration. Now let your 38-year-old self go back to your 33-year-old self. With all the wisdom and understanding of your older self, help your 33-year-old self understand" (Barnett, 1981).

"That's one reason why I left that job, they expected too much of me. I thought I would have more control as plant manager."

"Okay, remember this experience. You can come back to it whenever you want. Let yourself go back even further in time. Watch your life go by. Carrying your responsibility with you, be curious and wondering as you go back through time. Soon something will catch your attention. Let me know by lifting the index finger of your right hand."

Raymond lifted it almost immediately.

"Now, where are you?"

"I am at my dad's house sitting in the kitchen. My wife is at home. Dad is telling me about how I must be responsible for caring for my wife and eventual family."

"How are you feeling?"

"I feel angry. I have always been responsible. I did well in college and have done well since. He doesn't have to tell me that."

"Now, again let your 38-year-old self go back and be with your younger self. With all the wisdom and understanding of your adult self, help your younger self understand. . . . Now let yourself go back even further, watching your life go by, curious and wondering."

Raymond's finger lifted.

"Good, where are you now?"

"Again, I'm in the kitchen with my dad. I'm feeling angry because I'm about to go out on a date with a girl I knew during my first year of college. My dad is warning me about not getting her pregnant. I leave the room without saying anything. He yells after me, 'watch out!'"

"Okay, again, let your adult self go back and be with your college freshman self. Help him understand. Spend a few minutes with him helping him understand his frustration. Now bring all three younger selves together with your adult self. Experience the frustration of all three, and help all of you understand."

In future sessions we would go back even further in time, but here time ran out. Raymond had directly experienced his resentment of needing to be responsible and acknowledged its source: others telling him what to do. Raymond's openness to this experience reflected his gains in trust of the therapeutic process. The King within begins to clearly see the problem of frustration and responsibility and trusts the journey of the warrior within.

Megan, during a later session, her first without her husband, expressed resentment toward her husband. During their first session he was quick to define the family problem as her depression. Though she was cooperative during that session and learned something about her attempts to control her life and her need for her father to love her, Megan also resented "Doug's take-charge attitude and his telling the world I am depressed."

She began this session by saying just that. "He doesn't really care how I feel, he just wants me to always be happy and smiling. At work people accept me as I am. He always is trying to make me over."

"You couldn't say that when he was here."

"Yeah, he would have ignored me and run over me like a taxi cab in New York City. It feels hopeless to tell him how I feel."

"Okay, let's imagine Doug is sitting in that chair where he usually sits, and you just said what you said. What would he say?"

"He wouldn't have let me finish. He would have said he does care . . ."

"Say it as if you were him."

"I do so care how you feel, that is why I brought you here."

I put my hand up to cut him off and said "How does she feel? Give her a chance to finish."

Megan smiled, and finished. "You don't care how I feel, all you want is me to be smiles and happiness. It's impossible for me to tell you my feelings."

"Doug, now tell me in your own words what she just said."

Megan spoke for Doug. "I listen to your feelings. You are . . ."

Again I put my hand up and stopped Doug. "First, tell me what Megan just said."

Megan, speaking for Doug tried again. "You just said I don't listen to your feelings, but I do, you feel depressed . . ."

Again my hand went up. "Before you say how you think Megan feels, say what she just said and let's see if she thinks you got the point."

Megan laughed, "I don't know what he would do. He might just get up and walk out in frustration."

"If he were here that's just how the conversation might go, but I would let him know he could have his say as soon as you can verify that he understands what you had to say. If he got up I would reassure him that in a few minutes he could have the floor and that I would cut you off in the same way if you didn't take the time to understand him."

Megan left smiling, feeling I was on her side, trusting she was doing the right thing in coming to therapy. She planned to let her husband come again to the next session.

BEOWULF PROCLAIMS HIS PROWESS

Beowulf salutes Hrothgar, telling the King of his many exploits of killing giants and sea monsters. He vows to single-handedly deal with Grendel, requesting that he be allowed to purge Heorot of this monster. In just this way we need to "psych ourselves up" to meet the challenge. In therapy, the therapist needs to help "psych up" the client. Often hypnotic rehearsal is one way to motivate the client. The hypnotic rehearsal with Megan is an example of psyching oneself up to complete the task. With the trust of the king within and with her rehearsal of what she needed to do, Megan found the strength to follow through.

Megan and Doug came together to the next session, which went pretty much as we had rehearsed without Doug. Megan was quite self-confident in expressing her feelings, feeling the warrior within standing up. Doug did not attempt to leave.

Raymond now recognized the feeling of resentment caused by his driving need to be responsible. He had begun to face his tormentor and had a number of thoughts for a solution. Solutions were typical of Raymond's way of thinking. His first solution was to delegate more responsibility to subordinates, a solution presented him in a recent management training program addressing the issue of delegating responsibility. Raymond readily exhibited his prowess in preparing to attack his tormentor.

Craig, as you remember, worried obsessively about inadvertently saying something offensive at work through a memo or report. I asked Craig a question: "If you wrote something that would offend someone, what would you write?"

Craig thought a moment, "I honestly don't know. I never thought about it. It would just happen. I think I would write it without knowing or remembering I wrote it."

"But you don't know the kind of thing you might say?"

"I don't think so."

"Well, let's see if we can find what you might say. Sit back and relax. You had told me you enjoyed walking in the country. Imagine yourself walking along a country path. To one side of you are trees, a row of trees. To the other side is a meadow. It's a sunny spring day. As you pass through the shadow of a tree the air feels cool, and as you pass into the sun you can feel the warmth. Out in the meadow are wild flowers, butterflies, other insects busy working, animals. As you walk, enjoy watching the wildlife in the meadow. Your path is sloped downwards as you continue walking. As you look ahead toward the bottom of the hill, you can see in the distance a massive rock wall. As you walk, you continue to enjoy the warmth of the sun and the wildlife in the meadow, but your mind slowly becomes more preoccupied by the rock wall ahead of you. As you get closer, you are more and more amazed by the massiveness of the wall. It towers way above your head. You look to the left and the right—it seems to go on in either direction forever. When you reach the wall you turn and walk along the wall. Did you turn to your left or right."

"To my left."

"As you walk along the wall, you become more and more curious, wondering about this wall. You soon come to a door in the wall, a massive steel door. You try to open it but it won't budge. You walk further and come to another door. Again it won't budge. Soon you come to a third door and it is standing slightly ajar. You walk up to it and pull on it. You can open it a bit further, opening it enough for you to squeeze in. You look inside and see a long hallway with doors on either side. As you walk along the hall you find a door with a sign on it—'Craig's reports and memos.' You walk inside. What do you see?"

"Filing cabinets."

"Read the labels on the file drawers. Find the one that says 'secret memos and reports.' Place your hand on that drawer. Close your eyes. See what comes to mind."

"I see someone stopping me in the hall at work and asking me why I said what I said about him. I feel sick to my stomach. I say, 'someone else told me to write it.' I felt I was lying. I didn't know who told me but I don't remember doing it myself. He said, 'well it's not true, it's just gossip, I'm upset with you just spreading gossip . . .'"

"What's happening now?"

"I just had a flash of being in the hall at my high school."

"Be there in the hall of your high school. What's going on?"

"A guy I don't like is talking to me. He is the boy friend of a girl I like. I'd like to do something to break them up so I might have a chance with her. So I spread some bad rumors about him. She found out where the rumors came from. She hated me for that. She called me 'just a gossip.' I hated being called a gossip after that."

"Now let me ask you the question again. What might you say in a memo or report that would offend someone?"

"I guess it would be gossip, telling a story about someone that would hurt that person. I know gossip is wrong and I've prided myself for not being a gossip. I didn't think it was gossip about this guy. I just thought it was a way to show this girl I loved her, but I was jealous and it was gossip. I don't think I've ever gossiped since."

Craig now knew he was afraid to spread gossip, but he had made a commitment in high school to not gossip and he could not remember an incident since then when he did gossip. I asked him, "Is that commitment still alive inside you."

He answered, "Yes."

"Then you shouldn't be worried about spreading gossip. There may be something more you are afraid of. Feel the strength of that commitment within you, the strength demonstrated by your history of not being a gossip. Use this strength with curiosity and wonder, as you continue this journey over the next few weeks to learn more about your fear."

Craig left the office feeling great confidence that he had solved his problem. His understanding of the source of his commitment not to gossip gave him a sense of relief, and he thought he was over his obsessive worry. I wasn't so confident. However, I was confident that he would use this understanding to face the deeper problem, his deeper fear. Craig was beginning to show his prowess to overcome his tormentor.

Sometimes a person's strength is false, setting the person up for failure. Sally's enthusiasm and insight opened a potential door to failure. At the beginning of this last therapy session she reported, "I have a new male client who I know was undressing me in his mind. It's happened before and it's so disgusting. Yet I was able to let go of the feeling and not let it interfere with my ability to listen to his problems. Only with Bart does it upset me when I see his eyes watching me undress. Even though I should be able to be just me at home, I decided I could just ignore those feelings when Bart looks at me."

Sally was not married to her client. The relationship is different. She had higher expectations of her husband and her commitment to just ignore her feelings when Bart watched her dress was bound to fail. I answered her with the following hypnotic monologue: "We all have feelings—sometimes they are easier to control than at other times. You are right, it is important to control your feelings of disgust. You do it a lot. In the courtroom it is very important. If you are the prosecuting attorney you may want to express your disgust of the person you're prosecuting for the effect it has on the jury. If you are the defense attorney you may want to express compassion for your client even though you may feel some disgust, or if you are convinced of your client's innocence your compassion may be real, but in each case you are most effective when you are in control of your emotions. At home, though, with Bart you are more spontaneous and honest with your feelings. As you well know, at home you should be able to be yourself. You have high expectations of your husband, and in front of him especially you should be able to be honest. When you feel disgust it is hard not to express it.

"The real issue is not the expression of your feelings but the feeling of disgust. You know some women enjoy having their husbands eye them. It reassures them of their husband's love."

Sally was expressing her prowess. With this hypnotic monologue I did not want to diminish Sally's enthusiasm but did not want her to experience failure either.

Though her inner warrior was all psyched up, the king inside was wise and became aware of the potential failure.

HROTHGAR SAVES FACE

In his speech to Beowulf, Hrothgar recalls in greater detail his relationship with Ecgtheow, Beowulf's father. Ecgtheow had killed a man named Heatholaf, which had caused a terrible feud, leading Ecgtheow to seek sanctuary across the sea among the Danes. Hrothgar protected Ecgtheow by settling the feud with his money and treasures. Many years later, Hrothgar is experiencing feelings of hopelessness, as was Ecgtheow when Beowulf was a child. He is hopeless in the face of Grendel, to whom he has lost many of his followers and much of his wealth. At this time of welcome, Hrothgar appreciates Beowulf's confidence and inspiration in offering protection to his father's protector.

Because of the king's past protective acts, the warrior within has a debt to pay to the king and can pay it by slaying the monster. The all-powerful king has a way to save face by accepting the strength of Beowulf as repayment for this debt. The powerful king alone has the power to make decisions for the kingdom and to accept the help of this needed warrior. Though we recognize the great power of the warrior within, the wise king still occupies the throne, is still in charge, and the warrior needs to honor and respect the king.

In the examples above, I needed to reassure each client that the "battle" of giving up old ways of thinking is easier described than fought. I needed to reassure them that their depression, anxiety, fears, etc.—their adversaries—were real. The client's feelings need to be validated or "joined," for the client to save face—thus, saving face for the client's inner king. It would be easy to say, "You don't need to feel that way," but this response would only add to the power struggle by fueling the use of will power, and would not support letting go. Hearing "You don't need to feel that way," challenges the client to defend his or her feelings. Validating the client's feelings by offering face-saving words provides a mutual beginning point from which to move.

The most extreme example of the importance of joining the client is when a client is suicidal. By suggesting to the client, "Things aren't that bad, people care about you, you'll survive," the speaker is increasing his or her estrangement from the suicidal individual. The suicidal person then thinks, "You just don't understand." But when the therapist acknowledges, "You feel life is totally hopeless, no one understands, killing yourself seems like the only way out," using the language of the client, the client then can respond, "At least this one person understands." The king within is validated.

Last session, Aaron had found reason to blame his wife for his unhappiness. From the dream of "All I want to do is love you," Aaron realized how he relished the feeling of freedom of love in having an affair. He expressed some resentment of the burdensome nature of his marriage. This experience obviously was not leading him in the direction of being faithful to his wife.

The next session took another twist. Again Aaron came with a dream. "I think it was when I was about fourteen. I was at home taking a shower. There was some noise in the livingroom. I realized some youth of the church were arriving for my father's bible study. Most all the youth in the church were girls. I panicked because my father always wanted me to keep the bathroom door open a little so the bathroom would not get all fogged up and I thought one of the girls might come in."

"Okay, talk a little about your panic. What were you feeling more specifically?"

"Fear, I guess just fear."

"How about excitement. Wouldn't there be something exciting about one of the young girls catching you in the shower?"

"I don't know. I don't think so. I was more scared of my father and what he would do."

"How about guilt then. That feeling might make some sense too."

"Maybe. Maybe I should not have been taking a shower then but I didn't know or forgot about the bible study. I shouldn't feel guilty about the door being open since my father told me to leave it open, but I could never tell what he might say. He might have yelled at me that it should be closed this time."

"Okay, let's try on the feeling of guilt along with fear. What are you feeling afraid of and feeling guilty about now?"

"A day or two after our last session just before I left my office to go home I felt this panic. It hit me that I could not expect our marriage to have the freedom of an affair. How could my wife accept my need for this freedom. I guess that is no different from what we talked about last week, but last week I felt frustrated that my wife could not understand. This time it was panic, fear that I might lose my wife."

"How about the guilt?"

"I don't know. Maybe. I don't want to hurt her. She's a good wife and tries hard to please me. I don't want to lose her."

This commitment of his wife was a hopeful expression of his strength and prowess. This dream was an honest expression of his feelings of fear and potential for guilt. For a man to admit fear is often difficult yet feelings are difficult to deny in the context of a dream. Taking responsibility for feelings of guilt is also sometimes difficult but healthier than Aaron blaming his wife for making him feel guilty and thus resenting her. It was apparent that Aaron was not greatly in touch with his feelings of guilt, but this experience could provide him with greater understanding.

I continued, "That's interesting. Here's a thought. Last week you resented your wife for not understanding your wish for unencumbered love. Such resentment opens the door for a affair. This week you let go of that resentment and are more understanding and concerned for your wife. Now you are showing greater integrity by taking responsibility for your own feelings." These comments offered Aaron a way to save face from his fear by reframing it as integrity and a way to support or encourage the process of change. Introducing these comments with the phrase, "Here's a thought," left the comments open for Aaron to consider and possibly accept.

This language offered a means for the king within to save face, so that the king's authority could be validated—opening in the client a "yes-set," a phrase used by Milton Erickson (Erickson, Rossi, & Rossi, 1976) to describe a necessary mental set to induce trance. The client is answering each of the therapist's comments with a nonverbal or verbal "yes," a "yes" that validates the client's feelings or situation.

In our last encounter, Peggy was excited about her journey to find a forgotten memory. She felt assured there was a memory to recall, a memory of a room with amber light, a room with the shades pulled. Typically, people on journeys to find forgotten memories experience great anxiety about what will be uncovered. Because she has a long way to go, Peggy was not feeling anxious yet. Her defenses were in place and strong. She was more excited about being hypnotized. The amber light had two opposite meanings to her. She remembered the good feelings of taking an afternoon nap as a child and waking feeling rested, but, she stopped taking afternoon naps with the shades pulled quite a few years ago. She didn't remember when. She was always busy in school, and if she dozed off on the weekends, her spot was usually in the living room recliner. Amber light also triggered a feeling of nervousness, though Peggy thought she had no reason to be afraid.

I suggested we needed a safe place for her as a retreat on our journeys into the past, a place where the king within could protect her, a place to which she could consciously escape when anxiety or panic would overtake her. After a brief discussion, we decided the safe place would be her room in the home in which she grew up, an upstairs room with windows on two sides, both looking into trees in her own or her neighbor's back yard. I suggested that when we use her room in trance the shades be up. She offered no hints of anything anxiety-provoking that happened in that room.

"Sit back and relax. As you relax, picture yourself being in your room. Take a few moments to be there. What are you doing in the room?"

"I'm sitting on my bed."

"How are you sitting?"

"I'm sitting cross legged with my back against the headboard."

"Go on."

"I'm just looking around the room."

"Tell me what you see."

"I'm looking out the window into the tree in the back yard. There is a bird nest in the tree, and birds are coming and going."

"Okay, what is just to the right of the window?"

"My desk."

"What's on your desk?"

"Well, my school books, a jewelry box, a picture of my mom and me when I was small, and some bottles, and other stuff."

"Okay, go on around the room and tell me what you see."

"The desk is in the corner, then comes my bed, and a poster on the wall above my bed of horses running in a field. Next to the poster in the corner is the closet door. On that wall are several posters of horses and riders. Nothing else is along that wall except the door to my room near the foot of my bed. On the wall at the foot of my bed is my dresser and next to it is the other window that looks out to next door. There is a chair in that corner with a stuffed Winnie the Pooh sitting on it."

"Are there any curtains on the window?"

"Uh huh, light mint green."

"What is you bed spread like?"

"Green and yellow flowered print."

"What's on the floor?"

"Tan carpeting."

"Okay, sit there on the bed, relax, feel your mind, your body slowing down, listen for noises in the house. Do you hear anything?"

"No. I'm home alone. My mom doesn't get home until after five. I have an hour and a half after school alone. I like it. I like the quiet."

"What do you want to do, sitting on your bed?"

"I have my diary in the headboard of my bed that I write in most afternoons. I could write in it."

"Okay, go ahead and write in it if you like while I keep on talking. Sit there and relax. Feel the peacefulness of the afternoon. Enjoy your time alone. You know whenever you like, whenever you need to, you can come back to your room. Right now you can really relax and enjoy your room. During later sessions, when we are journeying into you past, or into anxious moments in you life, you can feel secure to know you have your room to come back to. Now relax, take five breaths. With each breath inhale calmness, and as you exhale, let that calmness go deeper within you. When you reach number five, you can slowly open your eyes and let your mind come back to the room, office, around you. Very good."

Though she now felt very self-confident, this exercise helped to prepare Peggy to face hypnotically possible trauma in her life with the assurance that she would have a safe place to which she could retreat. The wise part of her, the "king" within, maintains her authority on this journey, the authority to make the decision to seek a safe place.

UNFERTH'S JEALOUSY

Unferth, Hrothgar's most trusted warrior, challenges Beowulf's stories of prowess. He tells his version of Beowulf's competition with Breca and Breca's victory. Beowulf raced against Breca, swimming for a week in the open sea.

Unferth believed Breca was the stronger warrior and beat Beowulf to the shores of Norway.

Beowulf counters with his version of the story. He tells of Breca's fear in losing sight of Beowulf on this race. During a stormy night, fearsome monsters pulled Beowulf to the bottom of the sea, but with his sword, he was victor. He killed nine sea monsters, but he was separated from Breca. After this incident the ocean currents carried Beowulf to the shores of Lapland, much further than Norway. Beowulf continues by belittling the strength of Unferth, who has been unable to protect Hrothgar's kingdom from Grendel.

Again, Hrothgar is pleased with the stories of Beowulf's strength. His hope is growing that Beowulf will free him from the torment of Grendel.

As a therapist, I can expect a client to show some resistance in therapy, to fall back on old weapons, to look for assurance in old defenses, the jealous old warriors within. These old warriors are always there looking to save face, to maintain their power in what had been the tried and true path until they met Grendel, the tormentor our usual defenses could not defeat. These old jealous warriors need to be acknowledged and satisfied so that they can then defer to the power of the newly arrived warrior.

In journeys to uncover the forgotten, resistance is frequently encountered. Peggy, on a number of occasions in therapy, resisted facing the pain of her childhood trauma by retreating to the safety of her room. With patience and when she was ready, the barrier was broken and the forgotten uncovered. I answered her resistance with acceptance, recognizing her need to avoid the pain. With my acceptance, Peggy eventually gained the strength to reach back to the trauma.

Beowulf's telling of the story probably would not have convinced Unferth, but it was told for the benefit of the king within. Only when we are ready to learn about ourselves may direct confrontation work.

Aaron continued to feel more comfortable blaming his wife for loving him conditionally rather than blaming himself. He did not appreciate her nagging, her anxiety, and her paranoia of him having an affair. The ease with which he was able to blame her offered him an easy excuse to continue having affairs. Therapy was comfortable because, so far, it gave him more ammunition to blame his wife. Aaron resisted taking responsibility for his behavior. Still, joining the client in a supportive manner is the first step of overcoming resistance, and at least Aaron felt I understood his plight. He came to the next session complaining about his wife's nagging and paranoia.

During the first session of therapy I had suggested to Aaron that if every woman on this earth expressed her love for him, it still wouldn't be enough: he needs to love himself first. Though Aaron heard this statement, it provided him with only limited self-understanding. His laughter in response suggested he was not ready to accept the idea personally. Returning to this concept would provide him an opening to accept responsibility for his affairs.

The following hypnotic language was used without formal trance induction, a language that evoked the "yes set," a language that initially joined his own feelings of blaming his wife but then moved him toward greater responsibility. "You really hate your wife's nags and paranoia. You just don't know what to do with it. You don't want her to be upset with you, you want her to love you, but her nags and paranoia drive you away. It is so much nicer with the unconditional love you feel from your girlfriend. You would rather be with her. You feel so much heavy responsibility in trying to please your wife. You hate that responsibility. Wouldn't it feel so good if everyone could just love freely? Wouldn't it feel great if all women you met could freely express their love for you? Pleasing your wife is so exhausting. Your responsibility with her is so great and exhausting.

"Some men, though, seem to feel support and sufficient love in their marriages, enough love so they remain faithful to their wives. You just don't understand those men. Their lives would seem so boring, so empty. You need more love and excitement than those men, but what you need gets you in trouble with your wife. I wonder what those other men have that make their lives satisfying, something that you are missing. One thing those men have is they feel satisfied with themselves, they feel they are lovable. I wonder if, deep inside, you feel unlovable, if you sometimes wonder why anyone would love you. I expect, sometimes, that when others express their love to you, it is exciting at first, but it feels empty after a while. If you truly were able to love yourself, maybe then you could accept the love from others, from your wife, and find it satisfying."

As I progressed slowly through this monologue, I saw no indication that Aaron disagreed. As I spoke, my voice slowed down to match the rhythm of his breathing. He was in a trance, just listening, showing no resistance. Seeing that my pacing was adequate, I continued.

"I wonder what prevents you from loving yourself, what prevents you from truly accepting love from others, from finding their love truly fulfilling. From my experience, I find people who are unable to love themselves and accept the love of others grew up feeling that love was conditional. I think maybe we need to explore the love you experienced in your childhood and find a way to help you heal the wounds of feeling unloved."

This hypnotic speech came at the end of the session. After sitting for a few moments, silently, I stood up. Aaron stood up also, and we walked into the office area to check my appointment book. We made an appointment for the next week and, as Aaron was leaving, I said we would consider his experience of love as a child next week. His resistance to accepting blame was melting. Hrothgar's jealous warrior lost the argument.

Sally realized that in the professional setting, she could accept the looks her clients gave her, but at home she expected more respect. One minute she could be sexually or seductively playful with Bart, and the next minute, she could go into a tirade. She was not ready to change. What was the source of her resistance? The answer was in her dream about the rat in the clown costume, but I expected this answer was too threatening to face at the time. I ignored it. If you recall, Sally mentioned that as she held up her skirt in the dream, she had nothing on under it. I expected she was not quite ready to deal with her seductive or exhibitionistic side, even though she was the one who brought it up, and bringing it up could be considered seductive. I could have been wrong, but I played it safe or, in a sense, didn't let it seduce me. By ignoring her comment, I protected her from having to deal with it, and she didn't bring it up again.

Remembering this incident, I began an hypnotic monologue. "You are feeling frustrated. You are exhausted and confused. You have learned some things about yourself, and you felt good about what you learned, but you find you have not really changed. You are frustrated and impatient. Something else is going on. There is something else we have missed. I am wondering about other feelings you may have, feelings you really haven't faced. You feel disgust when men look at you. You feel disgust when your husband looks at you naked. You trust him enough to explode at him when he looks at you, but then you feel guilty for exploding. You make up to him by becoming seductively playful and he enjoys it. You let yourself enjoy it and you have fun together. You know you cannot explode at male clients when they look at you because it would not be appropriate, but you are disgusted anyway. They are being inappropriate. We learned these things from your dream about the rat in a clown costume. You felt good about what you learned. You believed, with this understanding, that you could change, that you could control your rage with your husband. The dream taught you a lot, but we are missing something. I think that something is something else you said in the dream, something you said when you were describing what the rat saw when it was looking up at you standing on the chair. You mentioned you had a feeling, a feeling you were wearing nothing under your skirt. Go back to that feeling. That feeling causes you some anxiety. In your dream you were wearing nothing under your skirt. Stay with that feeling. Let me suggest some words. As I say them see if they can be used to describe your feelings. Playful . . . guilty . . . dirty . . . excited . . . fun . . . disgusted . . . free . . . comfortable . . . embarrassed . . . seductive . . . rebellious . . . humiliated . . .

"Now, let your wise, intelligent adult self go back to be with you in your dream. Let your intelligent, wise adult self also consider those feelings. How would you describe your feelings?"

"All those words seem to fit in some way."

"What does your intellectual self think about those feelings?"

"I don't think I should feel guilty or dirty. I've prided myself on being a liberated woman—that's why my behavior bothers me so. I should be able to accept my body and enjoy sex. My parents never talked about sex."

"If they could have talked about it, or if you could have read their minds, what would they be saying?"

"Oh . . . I think they thought it was disgusting and dirty. Humiliating and embarrassing, huh. . . . I guess feeling that way is okay in some situations, but not at home with my husband. I'm not sure about seductive. When I get playful with my husband, being seductive is fun."

"What do you think when you see another woman who you think is being seductive?"

"I guess I think she is disgusting and dirty. I guess that's not fair, but I'm not seductive in public."

"Yet, guys see you as being attractive. You've noticed them noticing you. What does seductive mean, anyway? If they see you as attractive does it mean you're seductive?"

"I don't know. Guys just look at women, that's the way it is. And I just make a big deal of it."

"Yeah, it's just hormones, the way they're made. If they wouldn't look something would seem wrong. And women have hormones too. They have their own way of looking. That's okay. We each learn from our experiences in life to react to our own sexuality and the sexuality of others. It's a confusing and exhausting world of hormones."

I had opened the door to Sally's anxiety about her own seductiveness, left her with a suggestion that seductiveness is part of life, the way we're made. She considered the issue, first intellectually, and also with a sense of exhaustion and confusion, but at least, she considered it. Her—or my—resistance to talking about seductiveness (and exhibitionism) had been breached. Sally became more honest about herself—about her guilt, excitement, disgust and sexual freedom. The defense of denying her own seductiveness lost the argument before the king. At least the question was now in the open. Sally's liberated self had won the argument over her potential resistance, at least for the time being.

WEALHTHEOW NURTURES

As the laughter and cheerfulness of this celebration grows, Wealhtheow, the wife of Hrothgar, joins this company of men in the great hall. She is glad for their presence and passes a jeweled cup to her king and then to the men. When the goblet reaches Beowulf, Wealhtheow expresses her prayers that he will free the Danes from the torment of Grendel. She is greatly pleased with Beowulf's confidence.

The female archetype is very important in the development of a strong and healthy self. So far, we have grown in strength and confidence in preparation to face Grendel. This growth has been in our maleness, that part of us who acts, who does things outwardly, assertively, to or for others, in order to provide for, protect and heal others. Our femaleness, as will be examined further in Chapter VII, is that part of us that nurtures by bringing others to us, to receptively care for, protect and heal others. This receptiveness is also sensuous. Wealhtheow is the nurturing, receptive, sensuous part of us, a part that cannot be ignored or denied in our growth to be a complete person, a part of us that plays a much more important role than is indicated by her brief involvement in this ancient poem.

In opening the topic of Sally's seductive, sensuous, exhibitionistic self, I opened it with care and without making a value judgment. She accepted the opening without resistance. She has accepted her assertive maleness in her professional role in life. It is her femaleness, her nurturing, receptive, sensuous side, that is confused. She accepts this receptive, sensuous self to a degree intellectually, but she resists it at a deeper level.

Her receptiveness needs great support, needs the nurturance of Wealhtheow. Enjoying a bubble bath or a massage are two ways of accessing the sensuous self. I questioned Sally with regard to her husband's ability or patience to give her a tender nonsexual massage. If he were willing, could she accept from him the gift of a massage, could she let herself feel a massage as a pleasant experience? That was part of the problem. Massage, in her mind, was the preamble to sex. She didn't trust that he could give or would even understand a "nonsexual" massage. Sally admitted she is able to enjoy a leisurely bath, but she was unsure if she could enjoy a massage. I suggested she think about it, and possibly talk to her husband about it.

I offered her an hypnotic exercise to facilitate her sensuousness. "Sit back and relax. Imagine yourself lying back in the bathtub. Feel the warmth of the water. Relax. As you relax, turn your mind inward. Go on a mental journey through your body. Examine each part of your body to assess the amount of tension or relaxation. Often people don't realize they are tense when they are. Consider each part of your body. Appreciate those parts of you that you find relaxed. When you find tension, consider what you need to do to relax it, possibly just letting the warmth of the water melt away the tension, possibly moving, changing your position, possibly massaging it, possibly breathing relaxation into it. As you lie there in the bathtub, do what you need to do to relax even more deeply. Consider the bathroom around you. Is there something you can do to make the environment more relaxing? Would dimming the lights, lighting a candle, burning incense, playing some music make your bath more relaxing and enjoyable? Nurture yourself, feel the sensuous side of you blossoming. Relax and appreciate the way you feel as you take your bath."

Aaron also lacks the ability to be sensuous and receptive. He has received "love" in his series of affairs but does not accept it because he feels unlovable. He has needed throughout his life the nurturing, receptive love of Wealhtheow. His wife was able to offer such love in the past but had difficulty now because of her hurt and pain. When she was able to offer it, Aaron was unable to accept it, unable to feel the love.

In our next session, in examining the love Aaron experienced in his childhood, we talked most about what it was like being a preacher's kid and what the congregation of his father's church expected of him. He perceived many expectations, but he did not feel love. When he was being the good boy, the women of the church would ooh and ahh over him, but he hated that kind of attention and wanted to be outside running around. He remembered hearing other kids running and shouting in the park next to the church when he had to sit in the church quietly. He hated sitting there.

"I remember feeling trapped, feeling so hot and angry sitting there. My mother would hold my arm when I would move around. Her hand was so hot, my arm would burn, but I would just sit there looking down."

"Even now, when you think about it, you feel so hot and angry. You can feel your arm burning. You can feel the anger in the tension around your mouth." The tension around his mouth was observable. I continued, "Just sit there and feel your anger and tension, as if you could explode. You hear the kids in the park outside playing. On Saturday you would be playing with them, but now you have to sit there quietly.

"Now, let your adult self go back and sit there in church with your young self. Your young self asks, 'How much longer do I have to sit here?' Your adult self looks at his watch and says, 'About ten minutes. I know how long that ten minutes feels, it feels like hours. You don't want to be sitting there, you want to get out and play.' Just sit there with your adult self. How does it feel now?"

"That's funny—when you said that, I felt a breeze blow through the window next to me. I don't want to sit there, but I feel better."

"Stay with that feeling . . . Now, think about your adult life. Do you know any children in your adult life?" I ask, knowing he has no children.

"Nan, my niece, my sister's daughter."

"Tell me about her."

"She just started kindergarten. She's cute, always busy. I see her about once or twice a month when our families get together. What do you want to know?"

"That's good. When you are together, do you spend any time just with Nan?"

"Not really. She is always busy with other things and other people."

"Next time you are with them, just watch Nan for a while and put yourself in her shoes. Think about what she might be feeling with whatever she is doing. Then be your wise and understanding adult self and comment to her about how she might be feeling. For example, if she is picking at her food and doesn't seem to like what she is eating, mention to her, 'You don't seem to like peas,' or whatever she doesn't like, or maybe she likes her peas, comment on that too. Pay some sensitive attention to her."

This assignment is an attempt to encourage Aaron to be more receptive, more nurturing. It is an attempt to help him be to someone else what he needed as a child in order to feel loved. Whereas with Sally, Wealhtheow's role was to help Sally experience the sensuous side of herself, for Aaron it was to help him become more sensitive or nurturing to others, offering to them a new dimension in their relationship with their significant other.

Returning to Megan, our previous therapy session had been with Megan alone. Before that, Megan had come with her husband, who would expound at length about Megan's depression. In her individual session she was able to tell how Doug would not listen to her and how she had given up even trying to express herself to him. We proceeded to role play what the next session could be like with Megan expressing herself with my help. Megan felt validated and strong when expressing herself as she would like to do with her husband. Her assertive maleness was validated.

The next session went as we had planned. With some work we succeeded in getting Doug to listen to Megan's frustration. I supported her assertive role, allowing Megan to express her feelings and needs. Her need for considerable and continued nurturing from her husband was apparent, and the door for Doug to understand and fulfill Megan's need was opened a crack. With my assertiveness, Megan felt her feelings validated, nurtured by Wealhtheow. Doug eventually was able to restate to Megan's satisfaction, her feelings of frustration at his trying to solve her problems rather than just understand them. He then expressed his frustration at his inability to make her happy. This led to a brief hypnotic summary monologue at the close of the session.

"There are two ways of relating. One way is to do things for the other. The other way is to listen to and validate the feelings of the other. Each of us has different needs. Megan needs to be listened to and validated. Doug needs Megan to make his home a place of peace and contentment. When Megan complains, Doug feels the peace is violated. When Megan has feelings to express, feelings that triggers Doug's impatience, Megan feels violated. There is a place for both. If Doug could take a few minutes to listen carefully to and reflect on Megan's feelings, then Megan could feel peaceful and content in their home. Both Doug's and Megan's needs would be filled. Both Doug and Megan need to be nurtured and to nurture each other. This can happen with greater balance in both lives, the balance between doing for the other and listening to the other." The balance between the king and queen within.

The language of the "yes set," joining the client in his or her feelings, is the language of nurturance, the language of Queen Wealhtheow. It is the language of sensitivity, of reflecting and validating feelings. Wealhtheow needs to be well developed in a therapist and ultimately in the client.

70 / GRENDEL AND HIS MOTHER

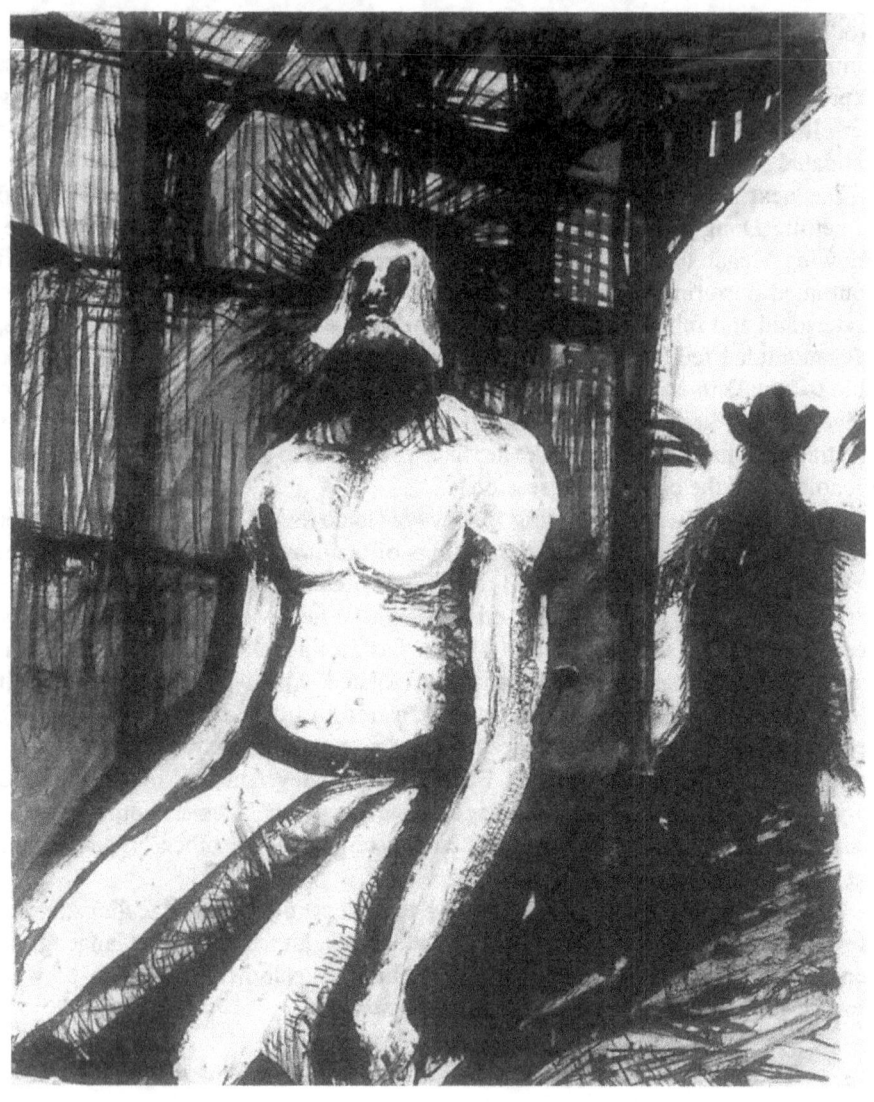

CHAPTER V

Beowulf's Preparation for Battle

King Hrothgar and the Danes leave Heorot for the night, entrusting the great hall to Beowulf and his men. The next several lines of the poem describe Beowulf's preparation to face Grendel. What are the elements of his preparation? First, the King leaves. Then, God is acknowledged as the sender of Beowulf to save the Danes. Third, Beowulf entrusts his armor and sword to a servant, offering a brief speech that he will not fight Grendel with weapons incomprehensible to this fiend: "Though these weapons could effectively kill Grendel, they will not be necessary." Fourth, Beowulf's men fall asleep anticipating the worst, that Beowulf will not survive the night. As the final element, Beowulf lays his head on his pillow, remaining awake, withdrawing into himself and allowing his internal fury to grow.

These five elements have bearing on therapy at two levels. First, they are the elements necessary in the process of hypnotherapy, and second, they are the elements necessary for a client to face Grendel alone, outside the therapy room.

HROTHGAR LEAVES, ENTRUSTING HEOROT TO BEOWULF

The King, the benevolent part of us, seeks to care for others in a compassionate manner. The King provides the people of his kingdom with a sense of security; so within us does our king archetype provide us with a sense of security in our interactions with our world. Usually we diminish our fear of the unconscious by structuring the unknown with our expectations of ourselves and others. The king's exit forces us to explore the unknown without the security and biases of our old beliefs and traditions.

Hypnotically, the phrase "with curiosity and wonder" sets the stage for us to face the unknown without the expectations that in the past have offered us structure and diminished our fear. The attitude of curiosity and wonder opens us to examine an unbiased unknown. Such hypnotic phrases as "what you find may surprise you" adds to our openness in facing the unknown.

The words "curiosity and wonder" facilitate dissociation in hypnosis, separating us from the king, from the distractions of our expectations. From the warrior's perspective, distractions can be dangerous. The warrior needs to act alone. The warrior within us cannot be distracted by our expectations, by our care for others or by our own self image at a time when we must single-mindedly face our enemy. We need to be left alone with the task at hand; thus, the king leaves.

Aaron exhibited an ability to dissociate, as evidenced in his ability to feel the breeze blowing through the window while sitting with his understanding adult self in the church. After this experience, Aaron began exploring the unknown or unexpected with curiosity and wonder. His undeveloped relationship with his young niece was another unknown to him, an unknown about which he was now curious and wondering. His focus of attention in life had been on women near his age, and he had been very self-centered. Aaron really had never given his niece any thought. At the next family get-together, however, he quickly discovered that just watching his niece caused her to run over to him with one of her books. He didn't have to say anything. He then read the book to her and she seemed to very much enjoyed the attention. When he asked her, "You like this book?" She quickly nodded and ran to get another. Aaron felt good about making a friend of someone he really had never noticed. Venturing into the unknown without his usual expectations or desires, he discovered how easy it was for someone to like him.

Megan and her husband, Doug, also had a therapy experience they were able to take with them and use at home—a new way to communicate. Though the old habits continued to arise at times, their new awareness helped them at other times to communicate more effectively. Doug's ability to listen allowed Megan to face her depression. Together they were venturing into the unknown, trying out new ideas, attempting to leave behind their usual expectations and desires—leaving the security of the king.

Sally came to her next session smiling. She had had a great time finding ways to make her bath more enjoyable. Though she had occasionally enjoyed leisurely baths in the past, she was generally too busy accomplishing things to let herself enjoy a bath. The only baths she could remember enjoying were when she was on a vacation or business trip, alone in a hotel at night with nothing else to do. She "splurged" one evening, locked herself in the bathroom with her CD player and a scented candle, to really enjoy the whole scene. When she finished, her husband looked at her and asked "What's going on?" She smiled and answered, "I was just enjoying myself." She ventured uncritically into the unknown and found it enjoyable, leaving her expectations, the security of the king behind. She could nurture herself and appreciate her sensuous side. A bigger step would be finding a way to include Bart in nurturing her.

When we last met Raymond, he journeyed back through time to three incidents in his life using the feeling of responsibility as the affect bridge. In the first incident, his boss called him to the office with the request that he work on yet another project. In the second he was newly married and his father was lecturing him on how he needed to be responsible. The third incident was when he was a college freshman and his father warned him about getting his new girl friend pregnant. Raymond felt angry and frustrated because his father did not trust him. Raymond experienced a degree of dissociation from his rational self in facing these three incidents. The king left, but the king's leaving was a matter of degree. We would go back even further in time with even greater dissociation.

During the next session we resumed the hypnotic regression. "Again, take your sense of responsibility back through time, being curious and wondering, as you watch your life go by. Go way back, go back to your early years, curious and wondering, carrying responsibility with you . . ."

Raymond was very ready to go way back. Whether as a result of the experience and practice from the week before or of something that happened to him during the week, he eagerly and almost immediately went into a deep trance, deeper than the week before. Without my needing to mention the lifting of his finger, his finger lifted.

"Where are you, what's going on?"

"It's the night before my first day in school. My mother took me shopping yesterday to buy me new school clothes. I was excited. That night I wet the bed and woke up scared. I pulled the sheets off the bed and stuffed them and my pajamas in the corner of the closet. I went to the dresser to get clean pajamas in the dark, couldn't find any but put on a clean pair of underpants. I laid in bed between the plastic mattress cover and a blanket. I was scared and uncomfortable."

"Okay, let your adult self go back and be with your younger self. Help your younger self understand."

"My daddy told me I am a big boy now because I am starting school. I was not a big boy to wet the bed. Daddy would be mad. I always try to be a big boy."

"Okay, now move ahead in time, to the next morning, the morning you are about to start school. What's happening?"

"Mommy comes into the room to get me up. She looks at me funny and asks me what is going on. I tell her I wet the bed and start crying. She holds me, and says it is okay, you were just too excited about going to school. I feel better but I'm still scared. 'Where's daddy? He's going to be mad.' She says he had to go to work early. She says she won't tell him. I hug her and feel a lot better."

"Again, let your adult self go back and, with all the wisdom and understanding of your adult self, help your younger self understand. Appreciate how understanding your mother is. Love her for it." I could see Raymond's chest heave in letting go.

When his tyrant king(s)—his critical self, his critical father, and the limiting king of his expectations to be perfect and in control—left, Raymond ventured into the unknown. On this journey, to his surprise he found the loving support of his mother when his overwhelming focus had been on the conditional, untrusting love of his father.

From a therapist, a client finds the emotional support and understanding he or she needs to face both the loss of his or her expectations and the insecurity experienced with this loss. But the client also needs to face Grendel when away from the therapist's office. In contrast to the security experienced in the therapist office, the insecurity felt at home and at work can rapidly escalate. For instance, Raymond might find growing insecurity when paying less attention to his usual needs of perfection and control at home and at work. As a result, a client commonly retreats to the security of old expectations after leaving the therapist's office. A deep hypnotic experience such as Raymond's can offer an individual greater confidence to face the unknown without the security of these old expectations. Leading the client to relinquish these expectations while the client is away from the therapist's office is another challenge of therapy that can be accomplished with hypnotic rehearsal.

Although Sally continued to struggle with her tirades that would occur when her husband watched her as she dressed or undressed, she had come a long way in understanding. She knew all along that there is something natural in men looking at women, but she felt a sense of disgust when men, especially her husband, watched her. She believed that when women tried to be sensuous, even seductive, there was something natural about it too, but she found such behavior repulsive and despised it in herself. She was now beginning to appreciate her femaleness by accepting and appreciating her sensuous side, but she was still unable to allow Bart to participate in her appreciation of her femaleness.

Sally needed to find a way to include Bart in her sensual life: the judging and critical king had to leave. When Sally returned next week she was eager to tell me of a dream: "When I was young I had a doll with a knob on top of her head. When you turned the knob you could make the doll have a sad face or a happy face. In the dream I was sitting on the floor with Bart in the playroom of the house where I grew up. I was holding the doll and Bart was just sitting there watching. When the face was happy Bart was happy and when the face was sad, Bart became scared. But what would happen is an arm, a strong arm, would reach over my shoulder and turn the knob. And the doll's faces were not the same faces. The sad face was a more frightened looking red face and the happy face was a made up, sexy face. I just sat there sort of like I was frozen, feeling scared or confused inside, maybe more because of Bart's reactions than the arm. Bart didn't seem to see the hand turning the knob but just the face changing. I guess I didn't either, I just felt a strong force turning the head."

I asked, "What else can you say about the strong arm or force?"

"I had no control over it. I don't know, I don't think it had a body but I didn't try to look."

"Okay, what part of you is not in control and strong?"

"I guess the part of me that panics, that screams at Bart."

"When you scream at Bart you feel out of control but it is a strong feeling."

"Yeah."

"Now, sometimes the Bart in your dream is happy and sometimes he is scared and confused, but he is really part of you. Can you find that part of you that goes back and forth between being scared and happy?"

"Yeah, that's the same part. I get scared and confused when I realize how angry I can get and how I scare Bart, but when I realize how angry I can get, I try to make up for it by making him happy by being sexy. When I am sitting at the table naked I feel like I am saying 'nyah, nyah, nyah, nyah, nyah, nyah' to the world. I sort of had the same feeling in the dream when the doll's face was sexy and Bart was happy."

"Wow, when you are sitting at the table naked you feel defiant, like you have strength over the panicky side of you. That's great you have that strength. Now, when you are dressing and Bart looks at you and you begin to get angry or even before you begin to get angry, sit down on the edge of the bed or on something wherever you are, partially dressed or undressed, and feel that strength of defiance come back into you. Share that defiance with Bart, let him be part of it, let him appreciate you. It may take some time for you to do, but be curious and wondering, prepare yourself, and when you are ready you will be able to turn your own head to see what that arm is attached to: you can see what is behind your panics."

Again, Sally had to do this alone, without the security of expectations, but the dream set the stage for the use of greater strength in facing her panic. Sally is the one who needed to sit down and wonder about her panic in a strong way.

Letting go of expectations is well described by Carlos Castaneda (*Tales of Power,* 1974) using his Yaqui Indian words of the *tonal* and *nagual.* In the world of Don Juan Matus, a Yaqui Indian sorcerer, the *tonal* is everything we are, everything we experience, our expectations and beliefs, everything we know. The *nagual* is that which is beyond the *tonal,* that which we have lost because of our expectations and beliefs. In our culture what we know, our *tonal,* is more and more restricted as we grow, restricted by our expectations. We lose more and more of our awareness of the *nagual.*

GOD IS RECOGNIZED—THE DIVINE INSPIRATION

After the king and queen and their band of men leave the great hall for the night to find their places to sleep, the word goes out that God has appointed a great warrior to stand up against Grendel, to protect Heorot and the Danish king. Thus Beowulf is recognized as divinely called or divinely inspired to protect. What is this divine inspiration?

God within us is our wisdom and understanding; God is our flashes of insight and inspiration. The psychotherapist talks through the client's God within by reframing comments and other hypnotic techniques that produce insight or the "aha" experience. These experiences of insight provide clients with the faith or knowledge that they will overcome Grendel. All doubt is lost to this faith. Facing

Grendel alone, without the security of the King, requires this inspiration. The two elements of the King's leaving and "divine" inspiration are inseparable.

Sally did not feel divinely inspired to find control over her tirades. But suggesting to her that her dream is a message from something deeper in her unconscious reframed her problem as something of great importance, as God-given or divine, thereby motivating her in her process of growth. My suggestion that she be curious and wondering as she looks to understand this message suggests that her tormentor is not destructive but is something to be faced and understood, even valued. Sally's acceptance of the strength of her agitation and indignation helps her to diminish her fear of losing control and gives her greater ability to look at the situation with wonder and curiosity. Reframing her reaction to her husband watching her as strength provides her with the insight and divine inspiration to face her tormentor with diminished fear.

As for Raymond, he uncovered his mother's unconditional love. Raymond's mother loved him even though he wet the bed. She knew that's what little boys do when they are excited about such things as the first day of school. Her unconditional or divine love inspired him to continue. Even though his father could be furious, she would protect him.

When Megan next came to therapy she reported that Doug had been trying hard to listen and she had been trying hard to care for him, but trying was exhausting and she had the feeling that nothing had really changed.

I suggested that since they were both trying, they both loved each other. I continued with an hypnotic exercise. "Sit back and close your eyes. Relax the best you can. Let your feet rest heavily on the floor and you legs rest heavily on top of your feet. Let your hands and wrists rest heavily in your lap and let your arms rest heavily on your wrists. Let yourself relax, sinking deeper and deeper into the chair. Relax heavily in the chair. Now, with your hands and feet feeling so heavy, *try* to lift your right hand."

Megan tried. Her hand trembled as she struggled to lift it but she couldn't lift it.

"Now *try* to lift your right foot."

Again she tried. Her foot trembled but she could not lift it.

"Trying is so exhausting and you get nowhere. The harder you try the heavier your foot and hand feel. Wouldn't it feel good to stop trying and just do it. Okay, just stop trying and let your hands and your feet relax. Let go of the tension, just let go. Let your arm rise and lift your hand from your lap. Let go and let your leg rise, lifting your foot from the floor. When you let go, things become much easier.

"You have been watching Doug *try* to become a better listener. His trying tells you he does love you. Feel that love. Let go and let yourself smile when you see him *trying* so hard to listen. Appreciate his love for you. Feel good about him, let go and do something for him. Take a deep breath and as you exhale let go of tension and feel a new energy flow into you. Go home and practice this exercise frequently."

Megan learned that the answer was not "trying" but "letting go." This divine insight gave her new hope, new energy to open up and face new issues, as we shall see in future sessions.

Peggy now had a safe room to which she could retreat when her journey into her past became painful. She also had her new boy friend and the beginning of a new life working as a paralegal in a new community, all giving her a fresh start and new strength.

At the next session Peggy was led hypnotically to carry her sense of panic and anxiety back through time. She began this journey with a sense of curiosity and wonder. Nothing special caught her attention as she went back to when she was seven years old. There she got stuck. During the session, she reported that she repeatedly thought about the age of six, tried to remember what happened when she was six, but she kept "bouncing back to seven." Everything she saw and remembered was when she was seven. She ran into a barrier. I suggested she picture a concrete wall cutting through her life at that age, and that her experience was okay. I suggested we could and would come back to the wall and eventually, soon, find a way through it.

At first Peggy expressed frustration, but I continued to promote curiosity and wonder, and continued to have great confidence that we would find a way through. The wall, I explained, suggested that "right now in your life, you are not prepared to find out what is on the other side. God (or your unconscious mind) knows what is on the other side, and God is protecting you. God has now told you something is there. You know that for sure. When you have the strength, when you are ready, you will find your way through. From my experience, it will not be long, maybe in a week or two, maybe between your therapy sessions, maybe in the next few days, or even hours, you will find your way through the wall. It is most important to look at the wall with great patience, curiosity and wonder, and what is on the other side will be opened to you."

Peggy's inspiration continued to grow over the next several weeks as she moved toward this opening.

During our last meeting with Craig we discovered he was afraid of getting in trouble for spreading gossip. His fear was traced back to a high school incident when he was caught spreading gossip in an attempt to facilitate the breakup of a girl he liked and her boyfriend. Making this connection, Craig felt confident that he understood his fear of offending someone at work. As a result of the high school incident, he had made the firm commitment never to gossip again, and to the best of his knowledge, he had succeeded. Thinking about gossip now at work seemed ridiculous. He was confident it would not happen. He thought he had his problem licked. His confidence was such that it seemed like a divine inspiration to him. I wasn't so sure. It seemed too easy.

Craig returned next session disappointed that his obsessive worry had not vanished. I said, "Sit back and relax. Close your eyes. You are frustrated because remembering the incident of high school gossip was not enough. There is something else. Be curious and wondering as we continue on our journey to understand. Let yourself again go back through time. Go back through time, back past high school. Be curious and wondering. Watch your life go by." The affect bridge is built or implied by mentioning the high school experience. "There is something else. Let each breath carry you back another season or another year, let each breath carry you back to an earlier event, person, place in your life, being curious and wondering. Soon you will come to something else important. What it is may surprise you. When you come to that something important, lift the index finger of your left hand to tell me you are there. Take your time as your breath carries you back." Craig's finger lifted. "Okay, come to a stop where you are in time. Let your breath guide you as you explore where you are. What is going on?"

"I'm at an old abandoned cabin in the woods. I'm with another guy, a friend of mine. I am standing in the door, watching my friend explore the mess inside the cabin. He finds a marble and puts it in his pocket."

"You're just standing in the door. How are you feeling?"

"I'm very uncomfortable. We shouldn't be there."

"What happens?"

"I say, 'Let's get out of here.' My friend looks at me funny but then shrugs his shoulders and we leave. We start walking back toward my house."

"Let the wisdom and understanding of your adult self go back and be with your younger self. Help your younger self understand . . ."

"I was taught we should always respect other people's property. We shouldn't have been there."

"You still feel uncomfortable about being there, you feel guilty. Imagine your son being a teenager. What if your son had come home and told you about finding an abandoned cabin in the woods, what would you have said to him? First, before you answer that, let me think, what might I have said if it were my son. 'I'm proud of you, you didn't go into the cabin, and you were honest with your friend by letting him know how you felt. I'm proud of you.'"

"That would have been nice. My dad would have yelled at me, 'You should not have been there!' I hope I wouldn't have yelled at my son, but I probably would have told him he shouldn't have been there."

"Hear inside of you your dad saying 'I'm proud of you.' That may sound strange to you if he never said that to you, but you can imagine it and feel it. 'I am proud of you.' Feeling that message inside of you, now go back to the cabin, stand in front of the cabin and consider what you feel and think."

"I would have felt good about my self . . . I may not have gone up on the front porch. I could have felt good about walking away. It might have been easier to say to my friend, 'We shouldn't go in there.' Dad did tell me he was proud of me playing football, and I loved playing football."

"Take a moment to feel within you these three ways it could have been said. Two negative, critical and one, positive. Feel within you the good feelings you would have had if your dad could have told you he was proud of what you did. Let that become part of your wise and understanding self. Imagine yourself telling your son you are proud of him. As you do, watch your son feel good."

This exercise provides divine inspiration. The "divine light" went on in Craig, you could see it on his face. He felt the strength and effectiveness of a positive attitude.

BEOWULF LAYS DOWN HIS WEAPONS

As Beowulf is about to bed down he entrusts his armor and finest sword to a servant, offering a brief speech that he will not fight Grendel with weapons incomprehensible to this fiend.

What are the weapons with which we protect ourselves? Our initial answer would include the many ego defense mechanisms written about in many psychology books: denial, dissociation, over-compensation, projection, rationalization, reaction formation, regression, etc. Beyond these defenses are our values, beliefs, and knowledge, or the lack thereof, that prevent us from recognizing the source of our despair and finding alternatives. Sometimes the lack of certain values, beliefs, or knowledge causes our despair and prevents us from finding a solution. Our experiences in life have been stored in our unconscious mind, but we may not have words for or the awareness of these experiences, clouding our understanding of the problem. Our narrow understanding or narrow mindedness provides us with what we believe are effective weapons, weapons that have been ineffective even though we have used them over and over. They are the only weapons we have known. We need to face our despair directly, with our bare hands, to find power over it, even though we may need assistance from someone skilled and experienced in understanding human behavior to help us discover the ineffectiveness of our usual defenses.

Earlier in this ancient poem, Beowulf and his men leave their weapons at the door of Heorot before they are escorted to meet King Hrothgar. This is the beginning, the first step toward trusting one's self and gaining self-confidence. As this story continues, the abandonment of weapons becomes more important as a sign of real strength and integrity.

The King's exit leaves us without the security of expectations, and our evocation of the God within provides us with the insight and inspiration to venture into the unknown. Now we can leave our weapons behind because we have found a higher and more basic or integral strength within us.

Craig's father's intent was loving, but he did not trust his son and believed that he needed to teach him right from wrong in a protective and critical way. Craig had internalized this need to protect and teach his own children in a critical or negative way. Though it is not simple to lay down such long term weapons, when Craig experienced how good it felt to be positive—to develop a sense of divinity rather than fear in a child—he was at the beginning of a new life.

Peggy believed she had suffered some form of trauma in her life but did not remember what. Her defense against this trauma was to distance herself, to dissociate from the trauma. She now knew something happened before she was seven, but she still did not know what. Her defense of dissociation was the weapon she needed to leave behind.

Megan learned that her weapon of will power, of trying, was not sufficient to bring about real change. She could change more effectively by letting go and changing the way she looked at Doug's attempts in trying to be a good listener.

Raymond returned the next week with a dream. "I was sitting on the ridge of the roof of our house with my wife, daughter and sons. Joan was holding Billy in her arms. There was a flood, and I was watching the water rise up around us. I didn't know what to do. I could see the tops of some trees in the distance but nothing else. The water reached my feet and then I woke, dripping with sweat and sick to my stomach. I laid there shaking. Thought I might be sick, the flu is going around. I took a few deep breaths and eventually fell back asleep. The alarm woke me and I lay there checking myself out. I felt okay. I was fine, got up and got ready for work."

"Wow, the ultimate responsibility, you needed to protect the lives of your family, and there was nothing you could do—no one, nothing you could rely on. It's still so alive inside of you. Even though your mother was understanding when you wet your bed, the importance of being responsible rests totally on your shoulders."

"Yeah."

"Did you have any physiology courses in college?"

"No."

"Well let me give you a brief lesson about the autonomic nervous system. I'm sure you already know a little about your nervous system, how nerves send electrical messages around your body telling the different parts what is happening and what to do. Well, one part of the nervous system is the autonomic nervous system, and it is divided into two parts, the sympathetic and the parasympathetic nervous system. The sympathetic nervous system governs the emergency response, and the parasympathetic system controls the relaxation response. If you are driving down the highway and some idiot cuts in front of you and you have to slam on your breaks, what happens? You heart speeds up, your stomach goes into a knot, your mouth goes dry, sugar comes from your liver and adrenalin from your adrenal gland. If your fear is great enough, you could wet yourself, your skin could become cold and clammy, or you might break out in a sweat. All these reactions are your sympathetic nervous system preparing you to react in an emergency. It's the emotionally reactive part of you. That's what happened in your dream. The panic of your dream triggered the sympathetic nervous system, preparing you for the emergency. When you took your deep breaths and began to relax again, your parasympathetic nervous system began to take over. It's the way you are made and your body was doing what it was supposed to do.

"Now there is something I want you to do this next week. When you get home from work and the kids are extra demanding, I want you to stop, sit down and listen to your body, see what your sympathetic nervous system is doing, check out your stomach, your chest, the rest of your body. Do the same thing at work when problems develop. Listen to your body, get in touch with that emotional part of you.

"If you feel an emptiness in your stomach or a tightness in your chest, or if you find some other negative feeling, think about your life when you lived in Philadelphia near your parents. You could share your responsibilities of life with them. When you lived in Philadelphia, you could easily drop your kids off at your folks', or talk to your dad about work. Now you can't do that as easily. Feel the responsibility or emptiness in your new life. Consider these thoughts and see how well they match the feelings of the sympathetic nervous system in your body. If they match, go over to your wife and give her a hug. Realize you are not alone. You share your life with another intelligent and strong adult. You don't have to be alone in your responsibility."

Raymond did what I said during the next week. He noticed a tightness in his chest, neck, and shoulders. Rather than being totally rational, he began to recognize his emotional side—at least rationally. But he admitted that he was unable to go to his wife and give her a hug. He didn't know why, but he felt uncomfortable giving her a hug when he felt anxious.

I then suggested, "Sit back and relax. Close your eyes. Take a few deep breaths. Let your parasympathetic nervous system take over. Follow your breathing. With each breath, inhale a sense of calmness, and as you exhale, let that calmness go deeper within you. Feel your body slowing down, your heart slowing down. Now, remember the evening when you last noticed the tightness in your chest, neck, and shoulders. Go back to that moment. Where are you in the house?"

"Sitting on a stool at our kitchen bar."

"Okay, sit there, feel that tightness, check out that tightness. Hear the noise being made by your children. Notice what they are doing. What's going on?"

"Joey is pulling at my pant leg, saying 'Daddy, Daddy.'"

"Reach down and pick him up. Give him a hug. What is your wife doing?"

"She is getting dinner ready."

"Look at her. Notice her breathing rate. Is it slow or fast. Look at her face, does she look relaxed or uptight?"

"She looks quite relaxed. She is breathing slowly."

"Good. Stay aware of how relaxed, self-confident, strong she looks. Now put Joey back down on the floor, or continue holding him if that feels good, and consider going over to Joan to give her a hug, maybe tell her you love her. What would happen?"

"She would ask, 'What's wrong?'"

"What could you tell her?"

"I wouldn't want to tell her because she is busy and I don't want to bother her about my problems."

"Really, okay, just in your mind, imagine telling her you feel anxious because you have so much responsibility. Just pretend you are telling her that. Take a few moments, examine how your body feels and then tell me how you feel."

"I feel even more anxious, my chest is tighter and my heart is going a mile a minute."

"A lot of men are afraid of using the word *scared,* but consider that word in describing how you feel." This sentence put Raymond in a double bind, giving him greater freedom to use the word *scared.*

"Yeah, it fits."

"Okay, now stay with that scared feeling and consider what you are afraid of. One possibility is that you are afraid you might disappoint Joan because you believe she expects you to be strong and responsible."

Raymond let out a sigh of relief, "Yeah."

When Raymond let down his defense of rationality, and accepted his emotion of fear, he felt a mild relief. I suggested Raymond go home and talk about this experience. He could open the conversation by asking Joan about how she manages with all her responsibilities in caring for three young children, letting her know he appreciates all that she does. Since Joan always asked how things went in therapy, Raymond felt he could talk to her about this experience.

When Raymond returned for our next appointment, he reported that he had talked with his wife about this experience even though it was difficult for him. He was pleasantly surprised when she gave him a big hug when he acknowledged all her work for the family. She then told of her appreciation for everything he does. Her appreciation felt good and Raymond sensed a load lift from his shoulders.

I suggested the same thing might help at work but not to expect hugs from his supervisors and managers. Raymond was able to laugh, realizing he might not feel the "great loneliness at the top" if he could express appreciation for the work of his supervisors and managers. Learning to express appreciation was a beginning to real change in Raymond's life. Because of his rational way of dealing with life, appreciation had not seemed important to him, nor did he think others needed appreciation. Now he knew that to receive appreciation he needed to offer appreciation. Raymond began to open himself to his emotional side. He laid down his weapon, his way of facing life with rationality, as he began his journey to find balance between the rational and emotional.

During the last session with Sally I suggested that when she saw Bart eyeing her she should sit down with a sense of defiance, partially dressed or undressed and with a feeling of curiosity and wonder, question why she should feel disgusted. Such an exercise can often provide some divine inspiration or understanding, but she was not prepared to stop her thoughts or feelings of disgust. Such patterns of thinking quickly become ingrained habits and are difficult to change. My suggestion was premature and I was expecting too much of her to stop in the middle of a rising feeling and sit down. Hypnotic role playing can help prepare an individual to change such ingrained habits. With an individual who is experienced in going into a hypnotic trance, an effective quick induction can be, "Sit back and relax. Close your eyes. Take a few deep breaths and let go of tension. Breath in calmness and exhale tension."

I then continued, "Let yourself be standing in your bedroom ready to get dressed for work. Where are you standing?"

"Between the dresser and the bed."

"Where is Bart?"

"He's still in bed reading the newspaper. He stays in bed until I'm out of the room before he gets up."

"Okay, take a few breaths to relax more. Know that Bart is going to look up from the paper at you, eyeing you as you undress. You are about to take off what you wore to bed. Think for a moment of different possibilities. For example, take it off more as in a striptease, seductively, maybe throwing it at Bart. Try that in your imagination to see how it feels. Think about these feelings for a few moments. Maybe stick you tongue out at him. . . .

"Now let's try another possibility. Go over to Bart before you start undressing and pull the blanket up over his head and ask him in a pleasant way to leave it there until your finished getting dressed. Again examine your feelings. Think about them for a few moments . . .

"Now take a few moments to think of other possibilities to try out. Try them and see how they feel . . ."

After a minute or two I asked her to open her eyes and come out of trance. I asked her about her experience.

Sally's first reaction to pulling the blanket over Bart's head was "That felt stupid, I'm no prude."

I thought for a moment that she was going to continue by saying "He has a right to watch me if he wants," but she didn't go that far.

She did continue "Throwing my nightgown at him and sticking my tongue out at him felt defiant and playful. We could both smile and laugh at that." She had not thought of any other possibilities.

"Okay, let's try another one. Close your eyes and relax. Your are ready to take off your nightgown and Bart is in bed reading the newspaper. This time as you undress, he ignores you. You keep watching him, expecting him to look up, but he keeps his head in the newspaper. Take a moment to let your feelings register . . . Okay, you can open your eyes and come out of trance."

"Wow, he can't win. All I felt was hurt that he was not paying attention to me."

"Go home and experiment in these ways. See what happens." This experience disarmed Sally. Though at home her habitual feelings would be more immediate, these other feelings would also be present and change her attitude about the situation.

BEOWULF'S MEN FALL ASLEEP

Beowulf is the most powerful among warriors. Though he has selected the greatest warriors among the Geats for this venture, they are not as great as Beowulf himself, for Beowulf was commissioned by God. They lack not only his physical strength but also his understanding and faith. These men possess the frailties of being human. Consequently, as they bed down for the night, they fear that they, and Beowulf, will not survive the night. It is a surprise that these men are able to fall asleep; yet, within us, in order to have the strength to face our tormentor, that part of us that lacks faith must similarly fall asleep.

We have within us two competing needs. First, because of our human frailty, we need to protect ourselves as evidenced in the activity of our sympathetic nervous system. We need to save face by maintaining our usual expectations and defenses. We have used them for so long that admitting their ineffectiveness now makes us feel foolish. Yet we have reached the limit of our frustration in dealing with our despair, and we are highly motivated for change. We have sought help, and to accept this help, we need to accept new ideas and let go of the old. Depending upon the confidence we hold in our therapist and the manner in which our therapist presents the new ideas, we are prepared to let our old expectations fall asleep and embrace the new. It is important for the therapist to avoid creating a power struggle with us. If a power struggle develops, we then rely upon our old defenses to protect ourselves from the therapist. The therapist, using hypnosis which necessitates the use of the yes-set, avoids a power struggle, allowing our band of warriors to fall asleep.

To avoid a power struggle as a therapist, I need to invoke the "yes-set"; that is, I need to pace carefully what I say to the client to insure that he or she is in agreement with me. I need to make statements to which I feel confident the client can answer "yes." According to Milton Erickson, the "yes-set" is the basis of hypnosis. It is trance inducing. For example, if a woman comes to me to quit smoking, a woman who has quit many times but always returned to cigarettes, I need to acknowledge she is very good at quitting, but each time she quits she begins to gain weight or she becomes excessively irritable, and therefore returns to smoking. To each of these ideas she can answer "yes," beginning the process of trance induction.

We have been inspired and we now believe we can kill Grendel, that which is tormenting us. Our inspiration gives us the confidence, in this case, to quit smoking. But we rely on our old weapons—we rely on our band of men who lack faith in the great warrior. When we feel nicotine withdrawal, we use the weapon of eating as a distraction to avoid facing the withdrawal. When we feel the nicotine withdrawal and feel agitated, we displace these feelings on our spouse or children. Our therapist needs to let us know these weapons are ineffective and that there are alternatives to eating or to displacing onto our children the agitation we feel because of withdrawal. With this assurance, we can let these weapons "fall asleep" and experience the faith that new ways will be more effective.

After trance has been induced through a relaxation exercise, I might continue, "Now, imagine yourself craving a cigarette. Examine the feeling you are experiencing. Some people describe this feeling as anxious, hyper, wired, or touchy. Spend a few moments to find your best word to describe the feeling. Now consider what is happening inside your body. Your body has had doses of nicotine many times a day for many years. Your body wants another dose, but you wisely are not giving it another dose. Your body is in the process of healing itself. Your feeling of craving a cigarette is like a cut: while it heals, it itches. You would like to scratch that itch, but you know that scratching might delay the healing process. You know in a day or two the itch will go away, so you simply put up with it. Your anxious feeling is like that itch. When you face it and accept it as a sign of your body healing itself, you can feel proud of the fact you are helping your body heal by not smoking. As you face the craving feeling, watch that feeling diminish. You know the feeling will be gone in a few days. You don't have to eat or become irritable, because you are proud of what you are doing for yourself, you are proud of becoming healthier. . . ." In this manner a healthy alternative is offered and over-eating or expressing irritability is lulled to "sleep."

For Sally and Bart, Sally's usual way of thinking and behaving, of feeling disgust and explosive rage, may not be asleep, but the intensity is diminished by the experience of the last session. She cannot help watching him while she dresses, realizing how she would resent it if he did not look up and how it would not be "her" to pull the blanket up over his head. Sally may have found the solution to her problem in this last exercise, unless there is a secondary gain to her behavior.

One potential for a power struggle to develop is when there is a secondary gain. If we, as clients, gain sympathy and dependency by maintaining our despair, or if we need to be sick to maintain our disability income, then we are highly susceptible to finding ourselves in a power struggle with the therapist. In this situation, the therapist needs to pay clear homage to our secondary gain by acknowledging it or putting us in a double bind with it. For example, Raymond's self image of a man was intertwined with feeling responsible for his family and with being strong and unafraid of this responsibility. When I mentioned that many men are afraid to admit they are scared, I put him in a double bind: for him to not be afraid, he needed to admit he was scared. If I had suggested Raymond was afraid of his responsibility, he likely would have denied this fear, and a power struggle could have ensued. The double bind lulled his fear to sleep.

Megan's relationship with her husband was improving with improved communication but, as you may recall, she came to therapy because of depression, because of a feeling of emptiness in her life. Because of her husband's growing sensitivity, Megan is now more able to admit and examine her depression. When I hypnotically led her down in an elevator, when the elevator door opened, she saw nothing. I suggested, "Look into that nothingness. What is it like?" As we proceeded, she described the nothingness as a small, cold, damp, black closet. As this experience developed she heard her parents fighting outside the closet. In that session, we began to deal with Megan's false belief that she should have been able to stop her parents' fight. She began to realize that her inner child needed parents to care for her and protect her rather than for her to protect them. She began to realize the inappropriateness of expecting a child to be the caretaker of her parents. Now she could provide support to her inner child.

Another issue with which we dealt in a later session was to face and reframe her sense of emptiness. Remembering the emptiness of the cold, dark, damp, and black closet, I asked Megan if she had something when she was young in which she put her important things, something like a box, drawer, or cupboard. She remembered a jewelry box she used for that purpose. She remembered that she had in this box, besides jewelry, the combination to her school locker, ticket stubs to events she went to with her boyfriend, and a love note from her boyfriend, among other things. I suggested she recall when she first received that box, when it was still empty. She recalled getting it for Christmas.

"When you first opened the package and saw the box, what were your first feelings?"

"I was excited, it was exactly what I wanted."

"You wanted something empty, a jewelry box, to put your important things in. What did you do with it then?"

"That afternoon I took it to my bedroom and had a great time organizing my earrings and other jewelry in that box. I set it on my dresser right in the middle. I remember looking at it just before I went to sleep that night. I loved that jewelry box."

"Remember the excitement of an empty box, the excitement of putting important things in it. Can you remember how your children would enjoy playing with empty boxes, sometimes even more than playing with what came in the box?"

"My kids always did like to play with boxes. They would do so many things with them—get in them, crawl around with them on their backs. Boxes are a lot of fun."

"Even though that closet you were in was empty, dark, and cold, how about the closets you have in your house now?"

"One thing we looked for when we were buying our house was the number of closets."

"Think of the opportunity, the fun of having empty spaces to fill. Think of the emptiness inside of you as something you are looking to fill. What fills that emptiness inside of you is the feeling of love. It feels empty because of the lack of love from your parents. You don't trust the love that comes from your husband and sometimes you wonder if your children love you. Begin to let their love fill the emptiness inside of you. Now take a few moments to see that love flowing in . . . . Now, let the love, the compassion, the understanding you feel for your younger self in the closet, flow in, let the love you have for yourself flow in. Take a few moments to feel that love flowing in . . . ."

Megan's fear of her emptiness was accepted and lulled to sleep, while Megan opened herself to the excitement of filling her emptiness with love.

The focus of Aaron's last therapy session had been on his recent family get-together. There he had ventured into the unknown without any specific expectations and desires. He found that he could relate to Nan, his young niece, in a friendly way and that she appreciated his attention.

At this point I developed an agenda for therapy, a strategy which sometimes interferes when the client has another agenda. In this case my agenda was useful. Aaron's feeling of a caring love, the care he showed to his niece, was warm, gentle, and healthy. His love affairs with other women had been exciting, intoxicating like a drug. These love affairs were addicting, like a drug used to mask his feelings of emptiness. This excitement was self-defeating because along with it Aaron felt a loss of integrity and, as a result, he felt even emptier. The caring love he gave his niece showed integrity and could eventually provide him with a sense of fulfillment, if he could learn to appreciate it.

If Aaron's "men" could "fall asleep," if they could give up for awhile their defense of excitement as a way to cover a feeling of emptiness, then Aaron could learn to appreciate the integrity of a caring love and find greater fulfillment in his relationships. His experience with his niece was a beginning. Thus, how could I provide Aaron with an experience to teach him the fulfillment found in a caring love, to provide a counterbalance to his need for excitement?

I began by offering him a hypnotic metaphor. "Sit back and relax; close you eyes. You are walking along a path. It's sunny out and you are feeling good. You have your in-line skates thrown over your shoulder, you're feeling carefree. You come to a fork in the path. One way is down hill and smooth. The other is up hill and rocky. At first you think, this is no decision. You're eager to put on your skates and fly down the hill. But then, the wise person within reminds you of your special ability: you can clone yourself and go both ways at once.

"One part of you begins to climb the hill. It is hot and you begin to sweat. The other part of you puts on your skates and, as you fly down the hill, the breeze cools you. As you climb the hill you can see the top ahead of you. It is wooded and looks cool. You look forward to sitting in the shade at the top. The other part of you continues to fly down the hill and you see in front of you a wide turn in the path. You look forward with excitement to flying around the bend. As you get to the top of the hill you come to a broad meadow with a stream flowing along the edge. You walk over to the stream, take off your shoes, roll up your pants, and sit on a rock with your feet in the cool water. You feel content and comfortable being in such a beautiful place. The other part of you flies around the bend to the bottom of the hill and into an oily swamp. There you get stuck and struggle to breathe.

"Now, sit back and relax. Come together and be there in the meadow, with your feet in the stream. You are there with your wife, sister, brother-in-law, and Nan having a picnic. The five of you are sitting around a blanket on the ground. There are wild flowers in the meadow and butterflies flying around. You feel content and comfortable, eating in a leisurely manner, passing the food around, tasting the flavors of the food and the smelling the scents in the air. Nan gets up and runs after a butterfly in a carefree way. You watch her and are able to appreciate the carefreeness of a child. You can feel that carefreeness yourself while sitting there next to the blanket and your family, a feeling you cannot feel when stuck in an oily swamp.

"You see a caterpillar and pick it up. It is crawling across the back of your hand. Nan comes over to see it and squeals. You gently put it on her arm and, as it crawls, she laughs because it tickles. You feel so warm and content, so peaceful. Now sit there and appreciate those good feelings, look at your wife, look at your sister in a loving way. Realize these two women understand you, care for you and are still there for you in their own ways, your sister in a sisterly way, and your wife in a wifely way. Feel their love in spite of your shortcomings, in spite of the part of you that is stuck in an oily swamp. Feel their love.

"Take this picture with you and visit it frequently throughout the day. Now take a few breaths, relax, allow yourself to feel good and content and gradually allow yourself to come back to this room around you."

This metaphor planted the seed of the fulfillment of a life with integrity, beginning to lull the other part of empty excitement to sleep.

ONLY BEOWULF REMAINS AWAKE

While his men are asleep, only Beowulf remains awake. He is preparing himself mentally, psyching himself up, for the fight, focusing his attention on his internal strength, alert to the world around him. In therapy this preparation is the mental strength gained through hypnotic rehearsal, rehearsal that the client is asked to practice many times a day.

In therapy, smokers are asked to repeat frequently throughout the day an hypnotic exercise of relaxation, of feeling the body cleansed by each breath of fresh air and, then focusing on the feeling or craving of wanting a cigarette: "Examine this feeling, find the right words to describe it, observe this feeling, and watch the feeling diminish." This feeling or craving is reframed by the therapist as the feeling of the body healing itself from nicotine. This exercise, when presented in the therapy setting and practiced by the client frequently throughout the day, is analogous to Beowulf's staying alert and preparing himself to meet Grendel.

Aaron's motivation toward living a life of warmth and fulfillment, feeling the love of his family, was growing: the warrior within was awake. The tormentor, his addiction for excitement, was there, too. He knew this addiction would lead him to an oily swamp, but if he thought of never having an extra-marital affair again, he felt depressed. Now, though, his image of fulfillment in life was a growing experience within him and offered him new possibilities of how to live.

Megan's preparation to face her Grendel was the exercise of remembering the value and opportunity of empty spaces, spaces that can be filled with important things. With this acceptance and understanding of emptiness, she faced her inner emptiness again with a new attitude of value and opportunity, filling it with love.

Craig continued to struggle with his anxiety and obsessive worry. Generally, his worry was a fear of doing something irrational that would get him in trouble.

Our last session had focused on his good father archetype. His relationship with his mother had not been approached. I sometimes ask clients to recall the phrases their parents used when they were upset with them. I generally offer examples, e.g., "I'll ground you," "after all I've done for you," or "you dummy." When I asked Craig this question, though he discounted its importance, he was quick to remember his mother saying not to him but to his brother, "Why can't you be more like Craig."

I asked Craig to imagine his younger self sitting in one empty chair in the room and his brother, Keith, in another. He described his younger self as "sitting straight with his hands folded in his lap, afraid to move." Keith, in contrast, "would not stay in his chair, was very impulsive and hyperactive, saying anything that came to his mind."

Considering these images, Craig was afraid of Keith, yet he envied him. "Keith was always getting into trouble but what he did always seemed kind of exciting. Keith, even today, seems to love life, but he hasn't done much with it."

I asked Craig to "spend some time each day, several times throughout the day, thinking of the things your brother did, the things that would excite you. Spend time thinking with curiosity and wonder about your brother in this way, especially when you begin to obsess about doing something that would get you in trouble, but think about him at other times too. Feel the defiance in Keith and the sense of defiance in yourself. Feel the excitement of defiance."

If obsessive worry was a result of Craig's need to be defiant, facing this feeling of defiance with curiosity and wonder could provide him with power over his obsessive worry. Regularly reminiscing about his brother's defiance and his own excitement would be a way of keeping himself awake in mental preparation to face his tormentor.

Facing the tormentor of obsessive worry generally does not provide the great fear that would be caused by facing anxiety or panic. Peggy came to therapy because of panic attacks. She experienced these attacks at night as night terrors or, in the morning as she awoke, as anxiety and fatigue. When I took her initial history, I questioned Peggy regarding her sleeping habits. She reported that she used to enjoy the experience of stretching out in bed at night to enjoy the coolness of the sheets and the warmth generated after a few minutes in bed. She now feels anxious when going to bed. Later, I used her earlier enjoyment of going to bed as part of a trance induction.

"Sit back and relax, think back to when you enjoyed going to bed at night. Stretch out and enjoy the coolness of the sheets and the warmth you feel after a few minutes in bed. Feel now that warmth and comfort. Lie there feeling relaxed and warm. Take a few deep breaths and with each breath feel yourself relaxing deeper and deeper, sinking deeper and deeper into the bed . . . Stay with this feeling of relaxation with curiosity and wonder. Be curious and wondering as you examine your feelings of anxiety and panic, the feelings you have experienced in your sleep and as you wake. Be patient, realizing this anxiety and this panic are messages to you from your body, from your unconscious mind, that something is bothering you. Be curious and wondering about the content of this message. Be patient as you wait for understanding. The answer may come quickly, or it may take some time. Let these feeling grow within you as you face them with patience and curiosity. Take your time. Practice this exercise many times throughout the day, just before you go to bed and just as you wake in the morning. When you wake at night, use this exercise as you go back to sleep. Be patient as you listen to your body for understanding."

This exercise was to become Peggy's mental preparation to face her tormentor, her anxiety and panic. This exercise kept her mentally alert and prepared to face her Grendel.

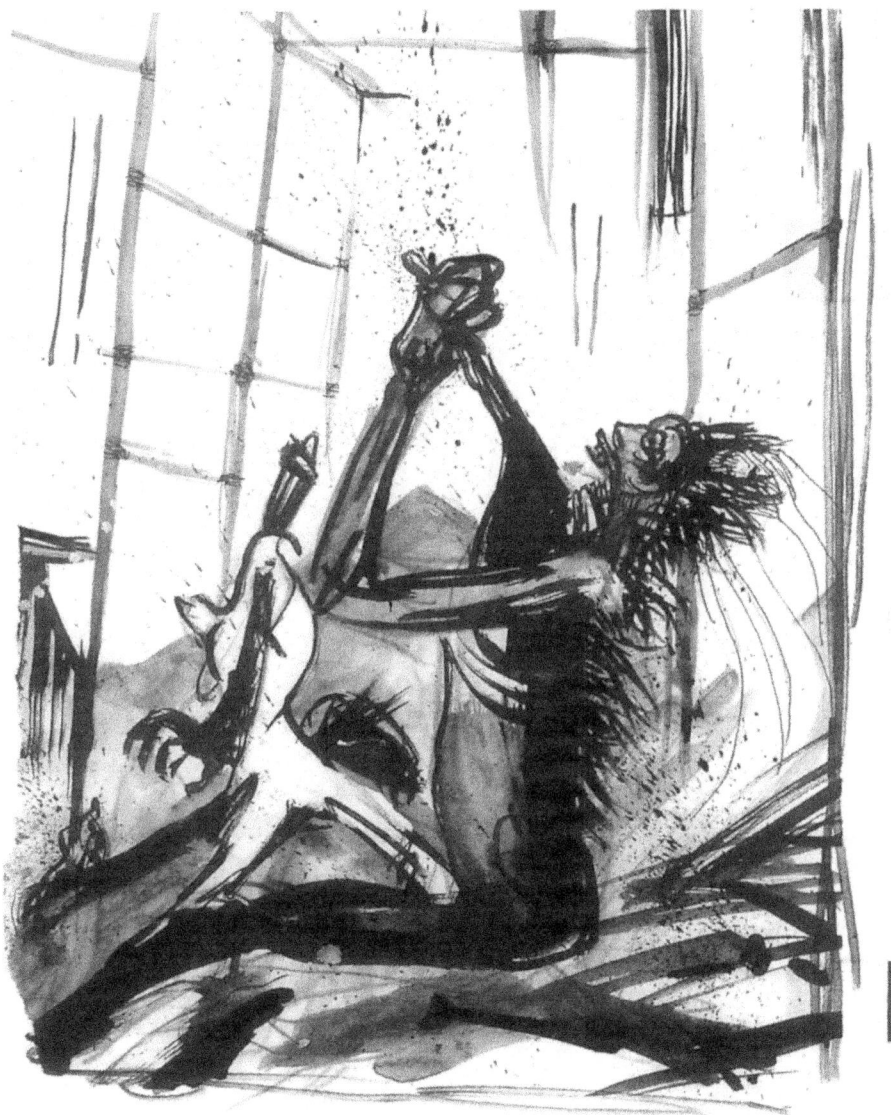

CHAPTER VI

The Death of Grendel

GRENDEL ENTERS HEOROT

Grendel Destroys the Door of Heorot

Grendel trudges out of the moors and finds his way to the great hall, intending to kill more Danes. It is not his first visit. When this unhappy creature finds the door secured with iron bars, he tears down the entrance with one touch of his claws.

Heorot, the great hall, is the basic structure that hold each of our parts, the structure that protects our archetypes. Though the hall is not destroyed, Grendel, as he enters, destroys its entrance, the focal point of its facade. Thus, he changes a central part of our outward appearance or behavior, our persona. Though we need to change internally, change our values and beliefs, our behavior and "appearance" also have to change. The question may be "which comes first?" Both generally change together, yet one of the maxims of Alcoholics Anonymous is "fake it 'til you make it." This maxim suggests that you must do the spiritual thing outwardly without waiting for a spiritual experience. If you simply wait for spiritual enlightenment it will not happen. When working with estranged couples, I frequently suggest a similar approach. "If you just wait for the feeling of love to return, it will not. But if you act in a loving manner the chances are greatly improved that you will recapture the feelings of love.

Craig spent some time thinking, both fearing and feeling the excitement of defiance. As a result, he recognized more vividly than ever his need to please others and his fear of confrontation and defiance. His thoughts of unknowingly offending someone were as close as he could come to living the excitement of confrontation, as close to his brother's defiance as he dared tread. He had a need to avoid being like his brother. He felt intimidated by any painful emotional energy. If his supervisor requested a meeting, he would feel anxious. Craig's self-image was of a person who felt intimidated by others and sought to please. His apparent success was because of his willingness to please others, but others often took advantage of him. He felt a loss of integrity when he would see incompetency or corruption and say nothing because such situations evoked his fear of confrontation. This loss of integrity would anger him, intensifying his need to defy and, thus, escalate his obsessive worry.

Now Craig was so disgusted with his people-pleasing self-image that he longed to destroy it.

Peggy practiced wondering with patience and curiosity as she lay in bed awake—wondering about the unconscious message of her anxiety and panic. As she did this she found a new level of strength. She sensed there was a message, something hidden in her unconscious, something that had happened of which she was no longer aware. She now knew she was about to uncover this something from its hiding place, and once it was discovered, she would be able to relax. Peggy now had a greater sense of self-confidence. Though she still had her night terrors, though she still woke anxious and exhausted, her attitude about her sleeping pattern had changed. Her morning anxiety and exhaustion had diminished. She was less terrified and more curious about her night experiences. Her excessive fear faded, allowing the portal to Heorot to be breached.

Sally was disarmed in the last session when she realized she would be offended if Bart ignored her while she was dressing. Yet, when she came to the next session of therapy she was nearly in tears. Though she had learned something her feelings hadn't changed. Again she had exploded in a rage, feeling disgusted when Bart looked at her with "those" eyes. She couldn't help herself. Her continued problem verified my thought that there might be a secondary gain to her behavior.

We continued with another hypnotic exercise. After a brief trance induction I suggested: "Go back in time, taking your feeling of disgust with you. Watch the events of your life go by. Be curious and wondering as time goes by."

After only a few moments Sally's eyes popped open. She looked upset. "I can't do it. I can't settle down. I feel just too wired."

"Okay, focus on your breathing for a few moments and with each breath, breath in quietness and as you exhale let the tension go. Realize that your unconscious mind is saying that you are not quite ready to know. But your unconscious mind is also saying that you are close to being ready, simply because if you weren't ready you would not be anxious. Anxiety is your unconscious mind saying that you are ready to face and overcome the problem. Traumatic things that happen at an early age are forgotten or repressed in your unconscious memory. As the years go by and your self-confidence in life grows, you eventually gain the strength to remember. This remembering begins with feelings of anxiety. Recognize in yourself this growing self-confidence. Just think how different you are now as a lawyer than how you were when you started law school, and especially when you finished high school and started college. You are now preparing yourself to remember, but you are not quite there. Face your rage, your anxiety, your feelings of disgust with curiosity and patience, knowing that you are moving in the right direction on this journey." Grendel had entered the great hall as Sally's increased anxiety and fear.

Recall that Raymond and Joan had formed a mutual admiration society in their appreciation for each taking responsibility at work and at home. This emotional support felt good to Raymond, yet he began the next session complaining about intense shoulder pain that woke him at night. His left shoulder was especially painful. Something more was going on, and he was ready to grab on to find out what.

I explained to him, "Sometimes things get worse before they get better. When you change using will power you are still the same person, but you have forced yourself to do something different. It takes a while for the change to become the real you. Notice your shoulders. You are holding them up. Let them go, let them drop. Let your elbows be heavy. Take your elbows off the arm of the chair and let them be heavy, allowing them to pull your shoulders down to a more relaxed position. Notice how much more relaxed your shoulders feel even though they still burn in pain. It takes a while for the pain to go away.

"Now take a few moments to experience the relaxation in your shoulders. Then imagine a yoke, like you've seen in pictures on the shoulders of an ox, resting across your shoulders. Imagine something hanging from each end of this yoke. Take a few moments to experience this load. One side is for your family. The other side is for work. Which one is on your left shoulder?"

"My family."

"Remember, that's the side that is hurting you the most." This brief experience may have been what set the stage or planted the seed for the important next session. Raymond's increased pain was Grendel entering the great hall.

Grendel Devours A Geat

Grendel enters the hall with fire issuing from his eyes. He sees Beowulf's men asleep on the floor. Wasting no time, he snatches up one of the sleeping soldiers, devouring him in an instant.

The death of this warrior represents the death of our usual defenses. We have remained dependent upon our usual defenses and also upon the part of us that lacks faith in our inner hero. Now, by destroying our usual defenses, defenses that are weak and meaningless, Grendel destroys our lack of faith. Paradoxically, though we experience a great personal loss, this act of Grendel actually frees us to face our tormentor with the real strength of our inner hero, Beowulf.

As mentioned before, whether in ourselves or others, we all have experienced many different defenses: denial, projection, rationalization, and reliance on will power, to name just a few. These defenses need to be destroyed. Craig's defense was his intense need to please others. This defense was flawed because of its ultimate impossibility, the impossibility of always pleasing everyone. Pleasing one person, after all, often means displeasing someone else. Craig's self-disgust for this image of being a people pleaser intimidated by any conflict or confrontation diminished the effectiveness of this defense. He was experiencing a need to be more defiant, to stand up for what he believed. His habitual defense needed to be, and soon was, destroyed.

Sally was mostly able to maintain an attitude of curiosity and patience as she let the Grendel of her disgust eat at her. She had the hope that she would soon find a solution. Similarly, Raymond was open to wondering why his family continued to be such a burden since he had shared his feelings with his wife and had gained the good feelings of her appreciation, yet the intense pain in his shoulders continued to eat at him.

Peggy was about to uncover a trauma in her early childhood. Its discovery would destroy her defense of dissociation from the trauma. Though she would still use dissociation at times, her awareness of this defense mechanism at least would give her greater control over it.

Aaron was venturing out to be a more responsible family man by getting to know his niece, Nan. Like most children, she responded well to his attention and he felt good about their growing relationship. But, in a broader sense, this new development did not mean as much to Aaron as did his self-centered need for the excitement of extramarital affairs. To Aaron there was still only one kind of love, Eros, the sexual, male-female love. He was not in touch with the fatherly love of relating to Nan

Something was really devouring Aaron as he came to the next session. He had had a dream that he could not get out of his mind. In this dream his relationship with Nan had become sexual. He knew that in no way did he have a sexual interest in children, but in the dream she was older. This dream frightened him and he was afraid to see Nan in the future.

I suggested that he redream this dream with my help. "Relax and close your eyes. Go back to the beginning of the dream, the picnic. You and Nan are just starting on your walk to the Rocks. Nan reaches up to take your hand as is natural for small children. She skips along beside you talking, telling you about her school. You soon get to the rocks. She turns her back to a rock and puts up her hands letting you know she wants you to lift her up on one of the rocks. You go ahead and grab her around the waist and lift her. She smiles and continues to tell you about the kids in her class. She has told you most of their names. She now mentions Dawson and tells you he is her boyfriend. You laugh and tell her that when you were a boy her age you thought having girlfriends was yucky. She laughs and says, 'I know, that's what Dawson says.' Again, like last week, this time with Nan feels good. She loves you but it is a different kind of love than you feel with an older woman. It is different from a sexual love. It is a good and healthy kind of love, kind of feeling, a feeling you are learning. There are many kinds of love and your feelings of love are growing, maturing in new and healthy directions. Take a few moments to experience the warm love you can feel toward Nan and let your appreciation for it grow. It feels good. Watch for other kinds of love in your life. Notice the love of the excitement of ideas you feel when you are talking about these ideas with other men at work. You feel another kind of love for these men. Let there be love all around you and all the time. Let these feelings grow as you go about your life this next week. A full life is full of all different kinds of love and all are exciting and full. One is no more important than another." Aaron left the session feeling better but I expect he still believed that sexual love was most the important and exciting.

Megan was depressed, feeling an intense void or emptiness in her life. An hypnotic suggestion has been planted that this sense of emptiness provide her with a personal opportunity, with space to be filled by something valued. Though initially this suggestion provided her with hope, as time went on Megan even more intensely realized that nothing really excited her in life, nothing seemed of real value. She had no real goals or aspirations. She enjoyed going to work because there she felt needed. On the other hand, she realized that her job was just a job, a way of surviving, leading nowhere. Her feeling of emptiness or depression intensified.

I suggested we return to that feeling of emptiness: "Sit back, close your eyes and relax. Go back to sitting in the dark closet. You feel an emptiness in the pit of your stomach. You feel a great void. You feel all alone. Hang on to that feeling for right now. Examine that feeling. The feeling has something to do with love or a lack of love. Bring the thought of love into the closet with you. You feel unloved. No one seems to care you are in the closet. No one seems to know where you are or even cares. You feel so alone and unloved. What you need is love. No one understands your feeling of emptiness better than your adult self. Your adult self knows your younger self better than anyone else. Your adult self knows you are in the closet, all alone and feeling empty. Find the sensitive and caring side of your adult self, and let that part of you go back and be in the closet with your younger self. Love your younger self. Your younger self is young and vulnerable. Your younger self needs your love. Your younger self is a sensitive and good young girl. She tries so hard to be loved. You are the only one who knows how hard she tries. You can go back and give her the love she needs. With all the wisdom and understanding of your adult self, you know how to love your younger self."

This time, tears came to Megan's eyes. She was able to do it. Whereas before she had found the younger-self disgusting and weak, now she had grown enough to be able to love her younger self. Megan could have set for herself all the greatest goals in the world, everyone on this earth could have told Megan they loved her, but unless she was able to first love herself, she would have continued to feel empty. Now her self-disgust was dying. Her need to gain the love of others through her deeds, her need to please her father in an attempt to gain love, was dying. Grendel was killing a Geat, one of her usual defenses.

THE DEATH OF GRENDEL

Beowulf Rises

As Grendel approaches, Beowulf rises to his elbow. Grendel knows he has made a mistake, but it is too late to run.

When we have lowered our defenses and we have found new strength within us to face and destroy our tormentor, then we are ready to withdraw within ourselves, to focus or direct our attention on the impending battle. Now we know we have the strength for victory.

Megan was now prepared to continue with the battle. She began to experience feelings of self love. Whereas before she had seen her job as just a job with no possibility of advancement, now she was able to find value in the positive feelings she gained from being needed in her job. She was beginning to see value in simple things, her energy was rising, she was rising to her elbow with greater self confidence.

The words of encouragement of different kinds of love lifted Aaron during the week between our sessions.

Peggy lay in bed curious and wondering. It was late fall and each morning when she woke it was darker. Russ, her boy friend, was working third shift, and Peggy expected him to come by after work. As she waited alone in her dark room, again a sense of panic came over her. But this time she had a flash, an image of a darkened room and a disheveled bed. This room and bed were in no house in which she had lived as far as she could remember. Though she was in a state of panic, another part of her realized that something in her life, a dark memory of something that had happened, was behind the panic. She knew at that moment that if she could remember what had happened she would find a solution to her panics. The picture and memory were very incomplete, but they were enough to convince her we were on the right track in therapy. Russ's love and her own new sense of self-confidence gave Peggy enough courage to face what she might uncover. She came to the next session with excitement and commitment. As the warrior within rose to her elbow, her Grendel pulled back in fear, realizing its demise was at hand.

Craig, who initially denied the significance of his mother's words to his brother, "Why can't you be more like Craig?" similarly realized, as he faced his feelings of defiance and assertiveness, standing up for his own ideas and beliefs, that his mother's words meant more to him than he thought. When he would have an obsessive thought of doing something wrong, the thought was of defiance, of intentionally doing things to "gum up the works." These thoughts occurred especially when he felt under pressure at work, when his boss asked him to do something extra or when he got behind in his work. The obsessive thoughts were clearly thoughts of defiance, and they were exciting. This realization came to him when he received an e-mail message in the shipping department asking him to come to his boss's office. Craig had heard a rumor of a change in plant procedures, and he knew this meeting had to be about this change. He had the thought of "accidently" erasing a computer file, an action that would create a real panic in the accounting department. All the way to his boss's office and during the meeting he excitedly obsessed about the idea. Yet at the same time, he was able to laugh to himself about the idea because this time he knew he would not do it. This new certainty was a relief. Craig now had the beginning of greater understanding. Now he could connect his defiance, excitement, and his feelings about his brother. He realized that his lack of assertiveness and his need to please others at the expense of his integrity were connected to his fear of being rejected as his brother had been rejected. In Craig's alertness to his own feelings, his Grendel saw the beginning of the end.

Beowulf Grips Grendel

Beowulf grips Grendel's arm and refuses to let go, a grip so tight that Grendel's talon cracks to bursting. The momentary realization of the client that he or she is on the right path provides the great strength not to let go. Peggy and Craig have Grendel on the run. Craig is flexing his new assertiveness and integrity.

Peggy knows she is getting close to uncovering some painful memory. I asked her, "Close your eyes. Sit back and relax. Be curious and wondering as you go back through time. Visualize the amber color of a room with the shades closed, blocking out the daylight. Let that color carry you back through time with curiosity and wonder. As you go back through time, soon something will catch your attention. When it does lift the index finger of you left hand to let me know you are there . . . ."

After some repetition of these phrases Peggy eventually lifted her finger. "I am in my girl friend's bedroom. We're sitting on her bed talking. It's after school and the school bus dropped me off with her. I had a note from my mother. She was busy and I wanted to be with Jill."

"How old are you?"

"I think I'm seven."

"Look around the room. What do you see?"

"The shades are closed and the room is darkened. Jill's bed is made and she has a stuffed dog on her pillow. She has several Barbie dolls lying on the bed and she is dressing one of them. I pick up one of the other dolls and am looking at it. It's warm in the room and I take off my sweater and lay it on a book on the chair next to the bed. The room smells good. She has a bowl of something sitting on her dresser, potpourri or something."

"How do you feel sitting there?"

"Nothing seems wrong. It seems nice but something in me says something is wrong. I feel uneasy."

"Listen carefully. Do you hear anything in the house?"

"It is very quiet. Jill's mother is doing something in the kitchen, but it is quiet."

"Let some time pass. What is happening now?"

"Oh! There is someone at the door. It's my mom. She stopped to pick me up. She is talking to Jill's mother."

"Okay, when she's ready, go with her. Sit in the car. Take a few breaths. Relax, comfortably let yourself come back to this office, and, when you are ready, open your eyes."

"That room felt like the room I saw last week, but nothing bad happened...."

"Well, we can always come back to that room. You have a better idea now of where it is."

Peggy grabs onto Grendel, she moves closer to uncovering her torment, but she is not there quite yet.

When we last visited Raymond he had realized that the load of his family was causing him more pain in his left shoulder than his work was causing on his right shoulder. Though he had always been a rational man, now he had begun to learn to listen to and experience his emotions. He could experience the pleasant feeling of being appreciated. Yet something continued to bother him. He was excited about therapy. He had changed, but he was also disappointed that things were still not great. Though he had not fallen back into his older pattern of irritability and explosiveness at work and at home, the tightness in his chest and tension in his shoulders not only had continued but had become worse.

"Sit back. Relax. Close your eyes. Take a few deep breaths. With each breath, inhale a sense of calmness and, as you exhale, let that calmness flow deeper inside of you. Examine your body, check out your feet and legs. Notice any sense of tension or relaxation within them. Your stomach, heart, chest, breathing rate, your lungs, your shoulders and neck. Continue looking for tension. Notice the tension in your shoulders. Take your elbows off the arms of the chair and let go of even more tension in your shoulders. Examine your neck. Feel the tension in your neck. Let your head slide back on your shoulders and bring your chin down. Though you may feel some tightness in the back of your neck, that position is a more relaxed and a more neutral position for your neck. In the long run, it will feel more comfortable in that position. Now sit there and appreciate the greater relaxation in your shoulders and neck.

"Now, though your neck and shoulders are more relaxed, remember the feeling of tension and tightness in your shoulders and neck. Take that feeling you remember with you and let yourself begin to go back through time. Watch the places and events, holidays and people in your life pass by as you go back through time, remembering the tension and tightness in your neck and shoulders. As you go back through time something will soon catch your attention. When that something catches your attention let yourself come to a stop in time and describe to me where you are and what is happening...."

After some repetition of these phrases, Raymond reported: "It was about two summers ago. Joey was about two years old. We were at a cabin in the Poconos and we were on a hike. Joan was carrying Joey on her back and he was squirming around. I had a pack with diapers and our lunch. Billy and Chris were walking. I realized how painful my shoulders were carrying that pack. The muscles were burning. I looked at Joan and she seemed comfortable with Joey on her back. I kept the thought to myself. I needed to share the load but felt irritated because I was in pain and Joan was not."

"Okay, let a few minutes pass; now what is happening?" I emphasized the present tense, since Raymond's use of the past tense indicated a lesser depth of trance. "What are you doing?"

"I see a fallen tree up ahead and I hurry ahead to sit on it for a few minutes until the rest catch up. I take off the pack with the excuse of wanting the water bottle for a drink. I think Joan is irritated with me for running ahead and leaving her with the children, who are starting to balk about walking. I think, 'why did we go on this hike anyway? The children are too young.' The others join me and we sit there. I'm so tense! I look at my watch and see it's too early for lunch. I'm ready to go back to the cabin but I'm afraid to mention it. I know in a few more minutes I will be carrying Billy as well as the pack. At least Chris believes she's too old to be carried; hopefully she'll start wining to go back. Then I'll suggest we eat lunch."

"You are carrying two burdens, the pack and your thoughts. Now let your 38-year-old self with all his wisdom and understanding go back and be with your younger self, help your younger self to understand."

"I suggested we go on this hike, because I know how much Joan enjoys walking in the woods. I wanted to please her, but walking isn't my thing, especially with the kids."

"Again you're carrying the burden of responsibility, the responsibility of making Joan happy. You've learned to share with her your appreciation but not your responsibility. You appreciate her and she appreciates you. Her appreciation of you is a great responsibility—it gives you a lot to live up to. On the hike you share the responsibility of carrying the pack but not the responsibility of your thoughts. You don't trust her with your thoughts. You believe they would disappoint her. Call the tension and pain in your shoulders responsibility. This next week listen to your shoulders, let go of that tension, let your shoulders down, share responsibility. Sharing your thoughts with your wife is a way of showing her your love. Letting her know you want to go on a walk with her because you love her and know she enjoys walks. Even though walking is not your thing, it is a way of telling her you love her."

A weight was lifted from his shoulders. "I didn't think of it that way."

Raymond told a brief story of ten years ago, when Joan's grandfather died soon after Chris was born. What she had to say he never forgot. She told him how much she had appreciated her grandfather because he could always listen to her and he would sometimes share his feelings. At that time Raymond felt envious and guilty because he hadn't been the greatest listener for Joan. He wanted his wife to appreciate him for being a good listener. Though included in what she said was that her grandfather would share his feelings with her, it hadn't registered until now that sharing feelings was equally important in showing love.

Raymond went home to tell his wife about the walk, about the thoughts, and about a battle he was having at work. He told her because he loved her, not because he was afraid of disappointing her with his burdens. He quickly discovered she was a good listener and did not attempt to solve his problems. She did not take on his burden. She did not need to solve his problems, because she had confidence in him. He was amazed that his problems did not seem to be a burden to her as her problems did to him.

In this discovery Raymond grabbed onto Grendel's arm and did not let go. How could he listen to Joan's problems and the problems of others at work without taking them on himself, but instead delegate responsibility and have faith that others could solve their own problems? He knew having faith in others and delegating responsibility was the right way. Though Raymond grabbed onto his new understanding, an intense struggle ensued, and he often regressed into his old habits. But when he did, the pain in his shoulder would remind him he was backsliding. His pain was a useful reminder that he needed to have faith in others and delegate responsibility.

Sally continued to fly into a rage when her husband would look at her "with those eyes." As hard as she would try, she could not stop her rage. She had the intent to stop and face her feelings with curiosity and wonder, but she would become incensed so quickly, she could not stop herself. She continued to feel a lack of control. The arm would reach over her shoulder and turn her head to rage. Bart continued to express great frustration with the situation.

Then she came to a session with a dream. "I was running. First, I was in our living room running on a treadmill, then I was running through town, then, all of a sudden, I was running out in the country. I felt like someone or something was chasing me, but when I looked over my shoulder whatever it was would dart behind a tree. I could see its shadow. As I ran I became more and more irritated, angry. I didn't know what was chasing me, nor did I know why I was running from it. Finally, I just stopped and turned around and yelled, 'whoever you are, cut it out!' I said it out loud and woke Bart. I could see the shadow behind a tree disappear."

"Tell me more about what was chasing you. What was it like to you?"

"It was confusing. It seemed like it wanted to hurt me, like it was angry, but I didn't understand why it hid behind trees like it was afraid of me. It was both angry and afraid."

"What part of you is both angry and afraid?"

"Oh! . . . I guess it is the part of me that goes into a rage, it feels like being angry about being afraid."

"Okay . . . Your rage is not just being angry at Bart for looking at you, but you are afraid of the look, and part of your anger may be at yourself for being afraid?"

"Exactly."

"How about when Bart looks at you with that look, you say to him 'you scare me with that look.' Do you think you could do that?"

Sally thought she could, that it would be easier to say "you scare me with that look," than to stop and wonder about it with curiosity. Sally was in the process of grabbing her Grendel. Even though she had been unable to stop her rage and grab her feeling, the struggle to do so had led her to the new understanding revealed in her dream. She had had a first victory over Grendel. Now she was prepared to grab on and not let go of Grendel. The next week she would succeed. Her new strength was the added understanding that her anger was at herself for being afraid.

Everyone is Seized in Panic

The hall thunders, and everyone is seized in panic.

The struggle with Grendel frequently causes a great turmoil within and with people around us. For Sally, her new strength minimized the struggle. The next time she felt Bart looking at her while she was dressing, she almost laughed when she told him "you scare me with that look." She had experienced a much greater battle those weeks before, when she wanted to stop her rage and could not, a battle that engulfed the great hall. Her regular inner warriors or defenses, the king within, and Bart were all seized in panic in the struggle. Now, with this new strength of understanding, Beowulf was easily the victor. Though we may anticipate an intense battle, a battle that brings us near to death, sometimes the battle is easier than expected, especially with the right preparation. The warrior had nothing to do but hang on.

Raymond was also lucky. He had his shoulder pain to remind him to not let go. The shoulder pain was that part of him seized in panic, his old ineffective warrior, his old habits or defenses in action. But, the warrior within knew well what to do to quickly bring order to the great hall. He needed to listen to and share his feelings with others. The shoulder pain could also be considered a divine message, a message from the God within.

Megan was able to reach out to her younger self in compassion. She was now able to show her younger self love, but both she and her younger self felt her emptiness together, thereby exaggerating the feeling of emptiness. This was seen in a dream she brought to the next session: "I was walking down the side of a dusty road with this young girl. We were holding hands. I think it was my younger self. It was like something I picture from the flat dry farmland of Kansas. Occasionally an old car would putt by. But we were alone, walking slowly like we did not know where we were going. We had no place to go. I didn't feel especially scared, just empty. When I woke I could still see this scene. I thought, what were they going to eat, or where would they sleep, but in the dream those weren't problems. I just felt very alone.

"It doesn't sound like you were in a state of panic."

"Only after I woke up and started thinking."

"Stay with that feeling. Don't let it go. It may be scary but it is important to face. See where it takes you. In your dream, though you felt alone, you weren't scared. You somehow had the confidence you would eat and sleep. You seemed to be ready to take care of your younger self. In your dream maybe it was just resignation but part of you was still okay. You had each other. Being alone is different from feeling lonely. Stay with the thought that being alone is okay." This exercise offered Megan a way to reframe her emptiness.

When we met him last, Aaron was left with the imagery experience that provided him with the warmth and fulfillment of different kinds of love. He began the week with the hopeful thought of experiencing love in many different ways, but then his wife expressed her feelings of insecurity and he felt the feeling of love rush from him. He wanted uncontrolling and unconditional love. With his "demanding" wife, love felt very conditional. He granted his wife the right to be upset with him, but this baggage was exhausting. Yet even so, his love was becoming more multidimensional.

I asked Aaron to characterize himself, his wife, and one of his extramarital lovers with the characteristics of specific animals. For himself, he felt needy, burdened and confused. What came to mind was a mangy mutt, wandering the streets without a home. His wife was frustrated, hurt, dependent, demanding, yet persevering. What seemed to befit her was a bloodhound—a dependable dog, serious, slow moving but persevering on the hunt. One of his girl friends was a flirt, carefree, spontaneous and bubbly. She seemed most like a miniature poodle: cute, bouncy, capricious, irresponsible.

"Now bring these dogs together in the vacant lot down the street. Watch them together. What do you see?"

"I'm surprised, neither the bloodhound nor poodle would have anything to do with the mangy mutt. He's so irresponsible, dirty, and ugly. The poodle seems like a floozy, with limited intelligence, probably the only reason why she would show any interest in the mutt. The bloodhound seems in a class by herself, far above the other two. I don't know why she is even there."

"Now, what would you like to do with these dogs?"

"I'd like to take the mutt and clean him up. He's disgusting. I wouldn't want to touch him though. But mutts often make, the best and most loyal pets."

"Can you find that loyal part of you?"

"Oh sure, I'm loyal. I would never want to leave my wife. I have never been interested enough in any of my girlfriends to want to marry them. My wife is intelligent, responsible, and the best wife and mother any family could have. She is the only woman I know who would take in a stray mutt."

"What do you want to be?"

"I want to be someone people, my wife, respect. I'd like to be a German Shepherd, strong and protective of my family."

"Take those images with you and work with them."

The following week Aaron talked of feeling strong and protective of his family, of feeling greater respect for himself. He saw one of his old girl friends and had an urge to talk with her, to attempt to seduce her, but his feelings were mixed. He felt disgusted by her and scorned his own thoughts. Yet he also felt the excitement of the potential pursuit and spent some time over the next two days fantasizing what could have happened. He felt some panic when he thought about the possibility he would never have an affair again. The panic reactivated his fantasy about the woman he saw. He felt partially proud of himself for his commitment to not have an affair, but he also felt disappointed because he was tempted, and guilty for considering and fantasizing about the possibility. Aaron was in a state of panic because he was still relying on his old defenses in his struggle against Grendel. But his task was to hang on. He had made a good start even though it was only a week. Aaron needed to hang on to his new image of himself as a reliable German Shepherd.

The Hall Stands

During Beowulf's tremendous struggle with Grendel it is a miracle that the hall remains standing. At the beginning of this chapter, the great banquet hall itself endures though its entrance is destroyed. Now, during the great battle, again the hall withstands the turmoil, but the benches inlaid with ivory and gold are turned over.

When Grendel entered Heorot, the destruction of the entrance represented a change in our outward appearance, or behavior. Now, during the battle, there are some inner changes, changes in our values, beliefs, and priorities.

In spite of Megan's panic about her dream, in the dream she found strength and survival. Her basic self still stood.

Aaron's behavior changed. He made the commitment to his wife to end his extramarital affairs. Internally he was still in a struggle, but his value to be a better person, strong and protective of his family, was growing and beginning to replace his feeling of emptiness and his need to seek empty love. The hall stood—his healthy values were being sustained.

Craig found some freedom from his obsessive worry when he could laugh at his impulse to "gum up the works" while realizing he did not have to act on it. By now, he had become more assertive with and able to question his boss. On several occasions in therapy we discussed meetings with his boss. I would assist him to find the most effective language to get his points across without threatening or intimidating his boss. Though he continued to be anxious and obsessive when he would seek an audience with his boss, he saw nothing to indicate his boss resented the interactions. He was surviving—the hall stood.

To reinforce Craig's success I offered an hypnotic ego-strengthening exercise. "Sit back and relax. Observe your breathing. With each breath notice your abdomen rise and, as you exhale, notice it fall. With each breath, breathe in a sense of calmness, and as you exhale, let the calmness flow deeper inside of you. With each breath, feel a sense of strength flow in and, as you exhale, let that strength become part of you. With each breath, feel a sense of self-confidence flow in and, as you exhale, that confidence becomes part of you. With each breath, feel the integrity growing inside of you, and, as you exhale, that integrity becomes part of you. With each breath, every day in every way, you become stronger, calmer, grow in confidence and integrity. You go about your daily activities in this calm, strong and confident manner. Your days pass in a relaxed and comfortable way. What had caused anxiety now is done with calm confidence. What had caused worry is now done with strong integrity. You are growing stronger and more confident each day in every way."

Sally found she could easily tell Bart, "Your look scares me." That phase defused her rage. It was a beginning—a beginning attained through willpower rather than attained with a change in her unconscious beliefs. The calmness didn't last. Sally thought she had the problem resolved, but after a few weeks she felt resentment creep in. Though she tried to ignore it, the resentment gradually grew until one day she again exploded. Both Sally and Bart were very disappointed, disappointment they expressed at her next session of therapy when they came together. However, I wasn't disappointed. I explained to them the false security of believing that the problem was solved. I reviewed and confirmed the facts that they had come a long way, found new security in their trust for each other, and were ready to face therapy at a new level. Their identities as individuals and their relationship were not destroyed by what appeared to be a step backwards. The hall still stood.

I suggested to Sally that she was "ready to find the name for the arm that reached over your shoulder and turned the doll's head."

When I mentioned finding a name, a name popped into her head—"Jake. I haven't thought of him in years. He was a weird guy in school, and he got suspended for several days for what he did. We were standing in the lunch line and he was right behind me. All of a sudden I felt his arm reach around and grab my breast. I turned and slapped him. We were quickly escorted to the principal's office and he was suspended. I was so upset, they called my mother at work and she came and got me. I don't think we ever talked or said a word to each other in our lives. I am not even sure now that his name was Jake. I totally forgot about it all these years. Huh, I don't think it means anything."

"But, that is very interesting. The arm reaching around and all. I bet he had been watching or looking at you for some time before that and, maybe, even after; why else would he do that to you? Maybe he was having some kind of fantasy about you."

"I don't know. It's possible. I have no idea what happened to him."

"Okay. Sit back and relax. Close your eyes. Take your time, but go back to the year in school when Jake grabbed you. It's a few days or even weeks later, and you happen to see Jake somewhere at school. Take your time. Be curious and wondering. You are walking in or somewhere near the school, and you notice Jake. Become aware of your breathing. Let your breath relax you and take you back to your school. Soon you will see Jake somewhere."

"Okay, I'm walking with my boyfriend out to his car. He is going to drive me home. I notice Jake just getting on the school bus. I ignore him but his head turns and his eyes follow me. I'm disgusted but I try to forget it, and I laugh about something with my boyfriend."

"For a moment, stay with the feeling of disgust. Let your adult self go back, and with all the wisdom and understanding of your adult self, let your younger self know you are proud of her, of her strength and values."

I could see tension leave Sally. She let out a quiet sigh. Over all these years she had been strong and self confident. She had fought a brief battle with Jake back in high school and thought she had won. Over all these years the hall stood but recently it had begun to shake in panic. Now it was ready to again stand steady.

The Geats Brandish Their Swords

In the din of the battle, the Geats wake. They draw their swords, the swords of their ancestors, seeking to protect their hero. They have no understanding that these weapons cannot touch Grendel. Our old and trusted defenses are still alive inside us. We continue to count on them, returning to them for validation when we are down. Our vulnerable selves return to the security of our old beliefs in the midst of change.

Sally had been brandishing her sword at Bart because of an earlier battle she had been carrying within, a battle she thought she had won years ago. She now faced her tormentor at a deeper level, an unconscious level, and made a connection with her history, the arm in her dream to the arm of Jake. She grabbed onto this knowledge, her Grendel, and did not let go. She is again the victor.

Craig reported a dream during the following session, a dream that illustrated the ineffectiveness of his defensive placations. "I was at the pizza shop I went to in high school with my buddies," he began. "The waitress brought the bill to the table. I grabbed it and got up to pay it. My girlfriend was sitting next to me and was smiling, but when I returned to the table it was my wife. She was collecting money from the others for their share and asked 'why did you do that?'"

"You paid for the pizza for everyone. What part of you would do that?"

"I wanted to please them, to impress them, especially my girl friend, but it didn't work. My wife thinks I'm foolish with money."

"Your wife thought you were foolish. What part of you feels you're foolish?"

"When I see something wrong I'm afraid to speak up. I feel I'm a fool for being afraid of standing up for what I think is right." Craig, brandishing his weapon, his defense of pleasing others, felt ineffective and foolish.

Megan, whose depression worried her husband, continued in therapy. She has been considering the hypnotic suggestion that her sense of emptiness was an opportunity, just as her empty Christmas jewelry box had been an exciting opportunity. Her attempt to find something of value to fill her emptiness at first simply clarified and exaggerated her sense of emptiness. When she was able to let her adult self love her younger, vulnerable self, she was able to begin filling her emptiness with the simple, caring things of life. Over the next month of therapy she reported two dreams.

The first dream occurred soon after her adult self found the ability to love her younger self. In the dream she was a teenager.

"My friends and I went to a pool party at a friends house. When we got there, Mel was not there and the pool was empty. We were disappointed. But, just joking around, we got in the empty pool and sat there talking. Then warm water started flowing into the pool and around us. It picked us up gently and we floated on it. It was a surprise, but it felt so pleasant. Then Mel came out and shouted, "Surprise, April Fools!"

"The rising water was not frightening but pleasant."

"Yeah, it was like water, but different. It was warm, didn't really get us wet. It was soft and comfortable. It's hard to explain. Maybe it was like a very soft comfortable mattress rising under us, but it looked like water."

"Okay, first you are with your friends and having fun, going to a party with high expectations. Then all of a sudden, you are in the empty pool, feeling empty and abandoned."

"Yeah, my feeling of emptiness came back even though I was with friends, but it was just there. We were talking and having fun."

"But then the emptiness was filled with something comforting and pleasant."

"It felt great. I was with my friends, and Mel then showed up so we were all together. I felt like I belonged."

"That's great, somehow in your life you are feeling like you belong, that you fit in."

"Uh-huh, my husband has been understanding and patient. It has been nice at home."

Megan was learning to look at the feeling of emptiness as an opportunity. As her fear of emptiness diminished, her tables of emptiness were upended.

About three weeks later Megan reported another dream. "I dreamt my husband was sitting up on the back seat of a red convertible, waving to the crowd, while riding in a parade. I was lost in the crowd. He didn't see me and didn't seem to care. He was not looking for me. I was upset and angry."

"Okay, first, what part of you is being honored in a parade?"

"Well, I have a full life. A job where I'm respected and appreciated, a good family, nothing is going wrong, and a comfortable home. I look at it and feel I should be happy."

"Okay, now, in spite of all that you have, you still are feeling lost and empty, and it makes you angry. Find that within you?"

"Yep, it's right there, the same feeling we have been talking about this last couple of months. It doesn't bother me as much, but last weekend my husband was invited to watch a game at a friend's house, and I felt left out and angry."

At moments when she least expected it, at moments of greatest vulnerability, Megan slid back to her old habits of dwelling on her feeling of emptiness, relying on her old warriors and their weapons. Yet she was beginning to gain some control over her feeling of emptiness, filling it with a sense of security and self love.

Raymond came to the next session in a state of irritation and impatience. "Why can't I just delegate responsibility and let go of all this tension. It just makes a lot of sense and I know it is good management but I still feel so much tension and a need to be involved in everything." He was brandishing his old sword of irritability, but this time more at himself than the others.

"You are delegating at work but you think you should not be as involved emotionally. You are doing it, but it takes sometime to let go of the feelings, to gain confidence in others as you seeing them living up to your expectations. But what is going on at home? Are you delegating more responsibility to Joan? That is something you don't want to do. That's different. Joan already does so much. She has her own responsibilities. How can you expect her to take on your responsibilities?"

"Yeah, I can't expect her to do more." I could see his shoulders lift.

"But there is something she can do that she is good at, something that most women are good at." Such statements that leave an individual hanging are trance inducing.

"What's that?"

"Go back to what Joan told you about her grandfather. What did she say?"

"You mean about how much she appreciated her grandfather because he could always listen to her"

"And?"

"He would sometimes share his feelings."

"What would she do with his feelings? She was only a little girl. If his feelings were heavy, what could she do?"

"I didn't think of his feelings being heavy. He wouldn't put them on her."

"Can you be sure? What do you think she would have done with his heavy feelings?"

"I don't know. She loved him. Maybe all she could do is cry for him. I can't imagine that."

"How about if her mother puts a heavy feeling on her, what does she do?"

"I don't know."

"Next time listen to her. I bet she says such things as 'Oh that's terrible,' or 'I bet that's hard to handle,' or other similar things. Generally there is little if anything she could do other than to listen with empathy, but that helps a lot. The other person feels understood."

"Yeah, I have heard her say those things."

"But you haven't given her a chance to say them to you. I wonder how such empathy would feel to you if you gave her a chance?"

The Wound

As Grendel struggles to escape Beowulf's grip, the sinew of the monster's shoulder snaps and a wound appears in his shoulder. Grendel pulls away, leaving his arm behind, and races out of the great hall. Beowulf is left standing, still holding Grendel's talon, arm, and shoulder. When we finally conquer our Grendel—Megan's emptiness or Aaron's extramarital affairs—he leaves mortally wounded, without his arm, the part he was using to destroy us. Still, we can't be sure he is dead. Sometimes the death of our Grendel is immediate, but more commonly, the monster's death is slow and anguished, as little by little we gain confidence that our agoraphobia, depression, obsessive compulsive behavior, etc. is weakened and eventually dies.

Megan's self love grew when she recognized the positive side of the little things in life, the understanding and support of her husband and the support she felt at work. As this self love grew, the wound in her feeling of emptiness grew.

Peggy had grabbed onto Grendel and had not let go. She had found the amber lit room, the room of her girl friend, Jill. During the next session we again used time regression to go back in time, and Peggy returned to Jill's room. Again, it was after school and Peggy's mother was busy, so she had a note to be dropped off by the school bus at Jill's. "We were sitting on Jill's bed and Jill's brother, Mike, came in. Mike is in the sixth grade. He wanted to play doctor. He wanted me to pull down my pants so he could examine me. I looked at Jill and she nodded her head. So I did . . . ."

"Let your adult self, with all her wisdom and understanding, go back and help your younger self understand how she feels."

"I don't know. I don't think he hurt me. But we heard their mom walking down the hall. Mike rolled off the bed onto the floor and hid. I pulled up my pants. She opened the door and asked how we were doing. We said 'fine' and she left. My heart was, is pounding. She scared me. I thought she was going to be mad."

"Again, let you adult self help your younger self understand."

"Maybe I was scared of what Mike was doing, it was wrong, but we were just kids and exploring. Kids do those kind of things all the time. I was more scared of Jill's mom catching us."

Peggy had found out at least part of what happened in that room. She felt satisfied that the unknown was uncovered; I wasn't so sure. But Peggy felt the victory of pulling off Grendel's arm. She hung on and in her mind, she won.

Sally spontaneously connected some weird guy named Jake to the arm that reached over her shoulder to turn the doll's head. Although she thought she had dealt with the problem back in high school and moved on in her life, that early "resolution" occurred through willpower, through the distraction of her boy friend without real, internal resolution. Jake's leer continued to reside in her. Now she has made the connection and grabbed on to it. Jake's leer was one look she could not trust. Now Bart looks at her in a similar way. She was engaged in a battle over whether or not she could trust Bart. In most ways she knew she could, yet that look triggered an old distrust.

At the end of the last session, I had recommended she say to Bart, "Your look is disgusting" rather than "Your look scares me." Again, she found relief for her rage. Saying this was now easy, and the two of them were able to laugh about it. She could laugh with Bart at herself. She had ripped the arm off her tormentor.

The pieces were gradually falling into place for Raymond. He had greater conscious control over his irritability, but he still let little things bother him inside. He knew his problem had to do with feelings of overwhelming responsibility. Though he recognized the need to delegate responsibility and share feelings, he still felt a great responsibility to care for and protect others. I offered him a metaphoric hypnotic experience during the next session.

"Sit back and relax. Close your eyes. Return to the heavy wooden yoke resting across your shoulders. It weighs you down. Hanging from it on the right side is a large bundle of your responsibilities at work. On the left side are your responsibilities at home. Responsibilities are of two kinds. One kind are the activities or things that need to be done—earning money, managing production, caring for and protecting your employees and family. The other kind of responsibility is more intangible—feelings of all kinds, feelings of responsibility for caring for and protecting family and employees. Look to your left and inspect your load. Look to your right and inspect your load. Know you can share these loads.

"Set down the yoke. Unwrap one side and pass out the contents to your employees. Unwrap the other side and pass it out to your family. Delegate responsibility. Share feelings. Stand back and be the real manager, the ring master, directing what is going on in each ring of your life. Feel the freedom of letting go and sharing responsibility. Sit back and relax and experience a new feeling of freedom."

The next week Raymond reported a dream. "I was again in the middle of a flood. Water was flowing through our house and I was running around grabbing everything I could and carrying it upstairs before it washed away. Sometimes I would have to run out into the front yard to grab something that got out the door. But the water kept coming up and I realized what I was doing was hopeless. Then I had a thought. 'What are all these things anyway?' I looked at what I had in my hand, some books off the book shelf and I just threw them in the water, smiling. I waded out the door, sat on the swing on the front porch, relaxed and watched the water flow by."

"Ahhh, freedom."

"Yeah."

"All the responsibility of possessions. You just let go of them. The earth is cleansing itself. So much unnecessary responsibility."

Responsibility's arm was torn off.

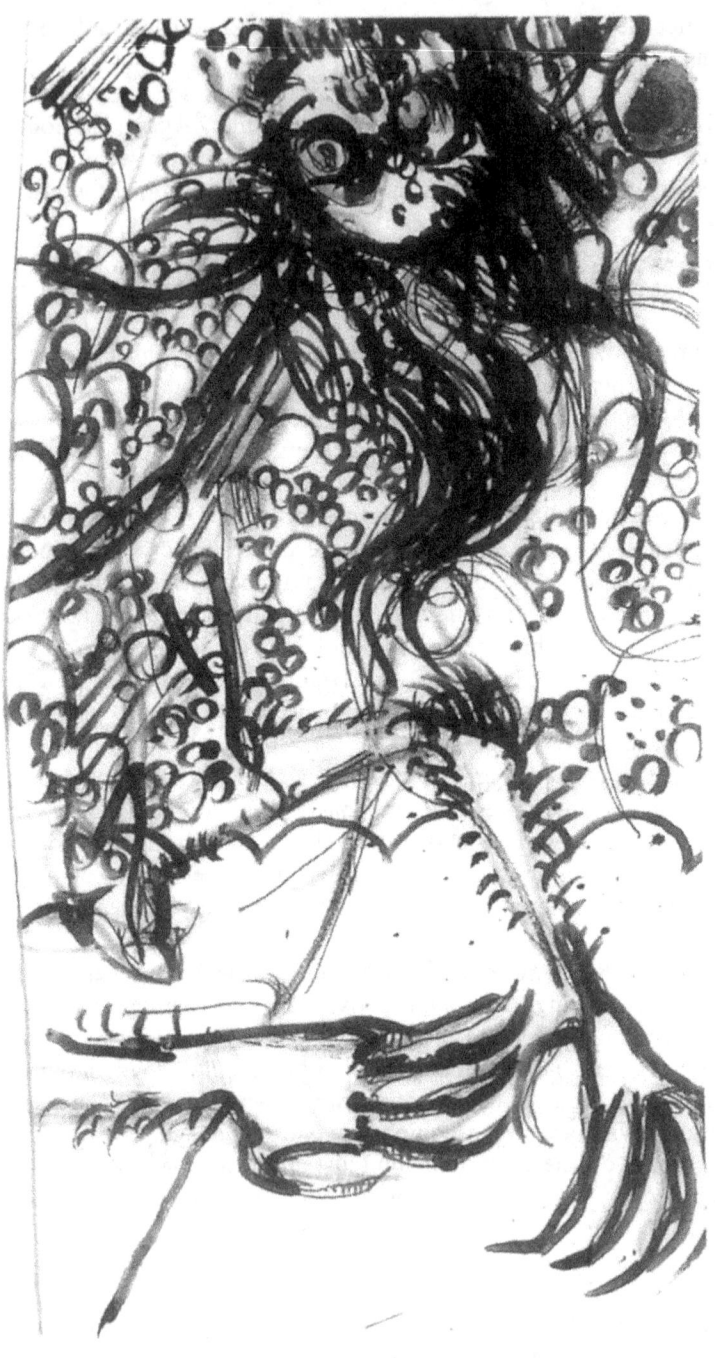

CHAPTER VII

The Celebration

GRENDEL'S ARM IS DISPLAYED

Beowulf rejoices in his night's labor and ensuing victory. He hangs the talon, arm, and shoulder, the full length of Grendel's reach and grasp, under the gables of the roof of Heorot. Similarly, our victory is outwardly displayed, a victory that radiates from us.

Each of the six people we have met in the last three chapters rejoiced in their victory. Each felt relieved from the torment of Grendel. Though Peggy had yet to uncover what was truly bothering her, she felt confident she would be able to deal with the lost memory when it returned. She was in no great hurry. She had the needed patience. Her anxiety was reframed as healthy excitement, an automatic reminder that she was on an exciting journey into the unknown, a journey she knew would bring her greater satisfaction in life. Her anxiety, reframed as a trophy of this journey, was hanging in the gables of the great hall. Raymond laid down his yoke of responsibility, felt freedom at a level deeper than he had ever felt, and was no longer bothered by neck and shoulder pain. I suggested to Raymond that he find some symbol of this experience he could carry with him. In his travels, he found at a souvenir shop a key chain with Paul Bunyan's blue ox wearing a yoke. This yoke was a reminder of his hypnotic and dream experiences, a reminder that worked to keep the experience alive within him. His key chain was the arm of Grendel hanging under the gables.

Sally related her feeling of disgust to an incident of sexual molestation when in high school. Now she was able to tell her husband of her feeling of disgust when he watched her dressing or undressing. In the context of her marriage this feeling now seemed ridiculous, and Sally was ready to let it go. The phrase "your look is disgusting," the arm of Grendel hung from the roof beams, was a reminder that "Jake" was now a thing of the past. Each person was able to rejoice and display some symbol of their victory.

Craig had been struggling with his obsessive worry, his fear of "gumming up the works" and his need to please others, especially his boss. He now understood his response to his mother's comment to his brother, "Why can't you be more like Craig?" This phrase kept him on the track of being good, of wanting to please "others." Yet his brother Keith seemed to have fun in his carefree life of being a free spirit, and Craig now understood that he envied this carefree attitude.

We also considered another influence on Craig, his father's critical and controlling nature. Craig's father's way of showing love was to be protective in a critical and controlling way. These factors were important determinants of Craig's anxiety, yet understanding them did not release Craig from his obsessive worry. Craig did not yet have Grendel's arm to hang under the gables.

Craig needed another connection to his past, which came from yet another hypnotic experience. "Sit back and relax. Again let yourself begin to go back through time. Be curious and wondering, carrying your obsessive worry with you."

Soon Craig lifted his finger. "Keith did something to upset dad. He had problems in school, and Mom and Dad had a special teacher's conference. He must have been in middle school, maybe the 8th grade. I think either Mom phoned his teacher or the teacher phoned home because he hadn't done some assignment. Whatever the cause, Dad is yelling at Keith. I'm in my room trying to do my homework, but I can't help hearing him yell . . ."

"Okay, go on."

"A door slams. I think Dad stormed out of the house . . ."

"Now, what happens."

"I hate this. I can't stand Dad leaving the house . . . I hear Keith's door open. Mom goes in. It's quiet. They're talking quietly. I then hear Mom say, 'Why can't you be more like Craig?'"

"Just sit there and let yourself hear 'Why can't you be more like Craig'. . . . Now let your adult self, with all the wisdom and understanding of your adult self, go back and be with your younger self as you sit in your room hearing all that is going on in your brother's room. Let your wise and understanding self help this younger self understand."

Craig wrapped his arms around his shoulders and bent at the waist. "I hated Dad getting angry. I think Mom did too. I think she was trying to comfort Keith, trying to get him to be good, so Dad wouldn't get so angry. I can see that silly expression on Keith's face . . . ."

"Tell me about Keith's expression."

"It's just silly, like 'why should I care?' I guess you would call it defiant. I'd have an urge to slap it. It just made things worse."

"Your mom was trying so hard to keep the peace. If she could have gotten Keith straightened out, Dad wouldn't have gotten so mad."

"Yeah, she meant well, but I hated to hear 'why can't you be more like me.' I feel sick to my stomach, it feels tied in a knot."

"You just feel tied up in a knot, tied up so you can't do anything. You have no freedom but to just do your homework and everything that is asked of you. You are so afraid to do anything else. You are safe when you're doing your homework. Feel yourself tied up. Again, let your adult self go back and be with your younger self all tied up. Your adult self knows your younger self better than anyone else. Only your adult self knows how your younger self feels. Your adult self knows the love your younger self needs to feel free, to be untied. Let your adult self show your younger self that unconditional love."

By now, a wet streak of a tear lined Craig's cheek. He was shivering. I let him sit for a few minutes.

"Now, listen to your breathing. With each breath inhale a sense of calmness and, as you exhale, let that calmness go deeper inside of you. Breath this calmness for a while.... When you feel calm, when you are ready, you can let yourself become aware of where you are and gradually open your eyes...."

This emotional release was the sign of Craig's victory over his tormentor. Grendel had lost his arm. The next week Craig came in with a sense of calmness. He hadn't obsessed at all during the week. It was a quiet session of review, reviewing the experience of the week before. I suggested he needed something concrete by which to remember what he had learned from that important session and his experience of the following week, something to hang from the gables of the great hall. Craig left with this assignment.

Things had been coming together for Megan. She realized she had much love in her life to cause her to rejoice. This love was seen in little things all around her. Yet she kept dwelling on her feelings of emptiness.

Christmas was approaching. Generally Christmas had become Megan's worst time of year, but this year her spirits were up. She was shopping in a different way, something we had discussed last session. We had used a role play exercise: "Pick one person you need to shop for."

Megan picked her nephew, Doug's sister's 9-year-old boy.

"What is important to him?"

She answered, "Dinosaurs."

"Okay, go to a toy store. Look at the dinosaur things, books, puzzles, figures. There is so much about dinosaurs. Don't buy him a lot. He won't appreciate it more. Buy him something small and simple. Being thoughtful is much more important. Make a list of each person you need to buy something for. Put next to their name something that is important to them. Buy simple things. The spirit is to be thoughtful, to think about them." This new attitude for Christmas shopping was the displayed arm of Grendel.

THE PEOPLE REJOICE

The people of Denmark begin to arrive to examine this amazing spectacle of Grendel's arm. They ride and gallop through the country side, enjoying without fear the freedom of their excursions. Similarly, in our victory we experience a new sense of freedom and carefreeness.

Megan's spirits rose as she shopped for Christmas, the perfect season to rejoice.

Raymond with his yoke also felt a new sense of freedom in telling his wife about the woes of being a plant manager, knowing that she would be emotionally supportive but would not take his burden upon her own shoulders. He learned he and his wife could share their emotional needs with each other, yet still be strong and responsible. He also experienced a new sense of carefreeness in listening to the trials and tribulations of his wife and children without feeling he had to always solve their problems.

Craig came the next week with a picture of him, his brother, and mother. His brother wore his defiant, silly grin and Craig looked very serious. He decided this was a picture he needed to carry. Though his dad probably took the picture, the fact that he was not in it represented to Craig his stomping out of the house. Another week passed without an obsessive worry. Craig was happy, feeling ready to rejoice.

Sally realized that Bart's look when she was dressing brought back all the feelings she experienced when Jake leered at her as he boarded the school bus. Yet she knew Bart was nothing like Jake, and when she would say to Bart, "Your look is disgusting," she knew she was confronting this tormentor within her and verifying that it was nothing like Bart.

Sally felt a new sense of freedom, of comfort without fear, when she was around Bart. She accepted his looks and began to feel attractive in front of him. She was able to dress and undress comfortably when he was present. Their need to be more "radical," like eating their meals naked together, seemed less important than before. Now was the time to rejoice, to celebrate.

I felt it was important to reinforce the couple's joy by donating something to their celebration. My donation was the suggestion they find something to memorialize the occasion. I suggested they go to a local art store and find an art poster they could frame and hang in their home. They selected not just a poster but an original print of a woman wearing a blue dress, sitting somewhat seductively on the floor in front of a mirror, with one leg pulled up with her arms wrapped around it. It portrayed an attractive woman who was able to admire and feel comfortable with herself, just as Sally could now admire herself and accept Bart's admiration.

About a month had gone by, and Aaron continued hanging onto his aspirations for being the loving protector of the family, the German Shepherd. He felt love for his extended family, his sister, brother-in-law, niece, mother and others, though he had not seen his father. This love was more than sexual and it felt good. His wife had noticed the difference—he was more involved with the family—and she told him of her observations. Aaron came into therapy rejoicing, believing he had his problem licked. In addition he had not been tempted by any woman, nor had he seen any women with whom he was familiar. Aaron had not had the opportunity to test himself.

TRACKING THE BLOOD OF GRENDEL

Some men follow the trail of blood left by Grendel, follow it to a murky lake seething with monsters and demons and boiling with blood. They return to rejoice the death of Grendel.

We need to verify the end of Grendel, the end of our torment.

Several weeks had passed before Sally and Bart returned for a therapy session. Their individual lives and life together flourished as they continued to experience their new sense of freedom. During those weeks they were very sensitive to any discomfort Sally might feel in her relationship with Bart, especially when she had to dress or undress in front of him. Her comfort continued. They had tracked the blood of Grendel and felt confident that he would not return. The weekend before their next visit they threw a party in celebration and enjoyed showing their friends their new art print, though they felt the meaning of the print was too personal to share, a sacred understanding to be held by just the two of them.

Peggy, to her satisfaction, had uncovered what had happened in the amber lit room. She, Jill, and Jill's older brother, Mike, were almost caught "playing doctor" by Jill's mother. She admitted she was more scared about getting caught than about playing doctor. I wasn't so sure that was the whole story; I felt it was important to track the blood of Grendel. The most sure way to find the assurance of his death would only happen over time, with the answer to the question, would Peggy again have night terrors?

I suggested another less certain tracking procedure. "Again, let yourself go back in time, back to when you were seven-years-old. Go back to Jill's room when Mike was there. Take your time. When you get there, lift the finger of your right hand. (Her finger lifts before I finish the sentence.) What is happening?"

"Jill's mother went down the hall to the bathroom and Mike quietly leaves the room."

"How do you feel?"

"Okay."

"How is your heart rate?"

"It's normal. I feel fine. We were just playing like kids sometimes play."

"Okay, now sit back, and picture a path going up a mountain. You can picture yourself at the bottom looking up the path, but also on top looking down the path, or you can be above looking down on the mountain and the path. Visualize the path. Some places may be smooth and not too steep, other places may be steep or rocky. The path may be very different in different places. Visualize the path. Now imagine markers along the path marking it in 28 equal sections, zero at the bottom and 28 at the top. Look near the top of the path, between let's say 25 to 28. How does the path look?"

"It's near the top and it is leveling off, not very steep. It's grassy on top."

"Now look at the path, between 15 and 20. How does it look?"

"It's steep. I can't see it. It is going through trees."

"Now look at the path from five to ten. How does it look?"

"It's rocky at the bottom, but from six up it is smooth though kind of steep. It's real rocky from about four to six."

"I forgot, how old were you when your parents were divorced?"

"I think I was two. I think my father moved out when I was one, but they were divorced a year later."

"And, you have never seen him since."

"Right."

"Your life was quite rocky until you were six?"

"Uh huh."

"The mountain path is fairly smooth between six and ten."

"Uh huh."

"What's it like from 10 to 15?"

"It's mostly smooth."

"Okay, continue to relax, and take a few moments to gradually open your eyes and become aware of where you are."

"What was that all about?"

"Sometimes people relate a path up a mountain to their life. Where the path is rough, times in their life are rough. Your path seemed most rough from the time your parents were divorce to when your mother married Bob. I was curious about your life before seven, the period of your life, that, a few weeks ago, you couldn't see or remember. You seemed to feel comfortable with it now though."

"Yeah, I've been feeling good about life."

Following Grendel's trail of blood did not support Peggy's sense of resolution that her problem was uncovered and solved. She had not explored nor had she expressed any interest in exploring any issues regarding her father or her parent's divorce. I suspected there was more to her night terrors.

Aaron made a decision to be the strong protector of his family and, in turn, he expected that his family would give him a sense of warm fulfillment and love. He wanted to give up the irresponsibility of an affair, but the excitement and unconditionality of the affair was hard to leave behind. He admitted he was loyal to his wife in that he never had wanted to leave her. He realized that he was vulnerable to temptation but also felt self-scorn when tempted.

Several weeks had passed. Aaron had had several encounters with both a past lover and the most recent one. The most recent girl friend continued to be available to him, but he had been successful in avoiding situations with her that would have led to sex. He felt good about himself, and with each passing day, his feeling of worth grew. His manginess as a mutt was healing. His coat began to shine. With each day that passed he valued his marriage more. The wound in Grendel's shoulder grew slowly. With enough time the arm would be hanging under the gable. Aaron felt he had attained victory. I felt less sure. I was in a bind: I needed to offer him the right balance between celebrating his victory with him and expressing skepticism. Too much skepticism would be the wet blanket to put out the fire of his victory, yet too much optimism would allow him to let down his guard, leading him to failure. While tracking the blood of Grendel, again he needed to be on constant guard, to stay on the right track, always prepared for Grendel's return. Excessive confidence in Grendel's death would set him up for failure. I offered Aaron an hypnotic metaphor to provide him with an internal safeguard.

Aaron plays golf. "You are on the golf course. You are having a great morning. Your confidence is growing. You're beginning to feel you can't miss a shot, but you've had experience with overconfidence in the past and know you need to avoid it. You know you need to keep your focus, but you're excited. Your excitement so well could cloud your focus. You deserve to celebrate your low score, but you are afraid you will quickly lose your lead if you lose your focus. You need to hang on to a healthy skepticism of your potential to win on each hole, until the end. In golf you have 18 holes, but life goes well beyond 18-weeks, months, years. Keep focus on your family, your values, your growing integrity to avoid losing your winning score."

A POET IMMORTALIZES BEOWULF

A poet, an expert with words, offers a poem to immortalize Beowulf. This poem compares Beowulf to the greatest warrior, Sigmund, skillfully paralleling the two heroes' exploits: exploits of rescue, of protecting friends and allies, of killing giants, and of gaining wealth and fame. The climax of Sigmund's victories arrives when he kills a dragon protecting a magnificent treasure. This treasure brings Sigmund great wealth. Sigmund was the greatest warrior since the evil Danish warrior-king, Heremod. The parallels indicate that Beowulf is appreciated more than the evil king was hated.

Immortalizing Beowulf in a poem moves the real Beowulf from reality into the immortal world of the unconscious mind. He is engraved in the minds of the people just as our new strength, the warrior within, is engraved in our unconscious mind.

Telling Peggy about the meaning of the mountain path, a metaphoric time line smooth between six and eight, immortalized for her an image of success in dealing with any anxiety or guilt regarding the incident in Jill's room. She wanted to believe her problem was solved, and this imagery reassured her she was right. However, I still felt something was missing.

Aaron's confidence grew. He struggled to maintain his guard. Finally, he let down his guard when his wife's confidence in his change became apparent. One day she told him how she appreciated his faithfulness. Her statement immortalized his victory. He wanted her confidence, and once he had it, he felt truly victorious. His guardedness was dangerously gone.

Megan had won her battle with Grendel but needed for her victory to be immortalized, to have a constant reminder that the simple things in life can be fulfilling. While Megan was sitting in the closet alone, she so badly needed her parents to miss her, to be concerned about her, to be aware of her pain, to show her they loved her. What she wanted from them was so simple, so little. As an adult she was now surrounded by such simple and little reminders that others loved her, but until now she had been insensitive to them and had not felt lovable. She needed something to immortalize this new understanding. She found a button that said "God Loves Simple Things."

I also offered her an hypnotic love-strengthening exercise. "Sit back and relax. Close your eyes. Become aware of your breathing. With each breath, as you inhale, fresh air enters your lungs, and as you exhale, the fresh air passes into your blood stream and flows throughout your body, cleansing and healing every cell of your body. Appreciate the cleansing and healing power of the fresh air. Appreciate the presence of the fresh air and your ability to breathe it. Appreciate those simple things in life. As you inhale, say to yourself 'I am at peace' and, as you exhale, again, 'I am at peace.' As you inhale, say, 'I am loved' and as you exhale, again, 'I am loved.' Feel the sense of peace and love with each breath you breathe. Look around you. Look for the sense of peace and love in what you see. Listen to the world around you. Listen for the sense of peace and love in what you hear. Smell the world around you. Smell for the sense of peace and love in what you smell. Find peace and love in everything around you."

Raymond experienced victory, too. He held a new sense of freedom in his ability to delegate both tangible and intangible responsibilities. He trusted his employees more with their duties. He shared with certain employees his concerns and struggles with decision making, and he found that he could trust these employees to provide meaningful and important input. He trusted Joan more with his feelings and concerns. The more he delegated and the more he trusted, the more he discovered he could trust and delegate. He found a new freedom in life.

The blue ox wearing a yoke was a useful reminder to facilitate this change in Raymond's life. Now, this change needed to be immortalized, needed to be accepted as a real part of him, needed to be fixed in his unconscious mind. This new self was immortalized in a dream. "I had a strange dream, all it was was gears spinning. One large gear was turning several small gears, turning about ten times faster than the large gear. On the shafts of each small gear was another large gear that was turning several small gears, each turning about a hundred times faster than the first gear. On the shafts of each of these small gears was another large gear that, again, was turning several small gears. These small gears were turning a thousand times faster than the first gear. This went on and on. That's all there was to the dream, gears spinning."

"Wow, just one gear turning all these other gears faster and faster. At one end a gear is working, turning slowly. At the other end many other gears are turning much faster. What part of you is the slow gear turning all the other gears, making them go faster and faster?"

"That must be my job as a plant manager."

"How does it feel to be turning all those other gears?"

"Fine, it just happens, the gears are turning just like they are suppose to turn. My job is to just keep them turning."

"Okay, the many gears at the other end are spinning much faster. What part of you are those gears?"

"They're not me but all the people who work in the plant."

"But you turn them, and you are all part of the whole needed to produce your widgets, you are part of the whole, all parts are necessary. You are necessary to keep things going. You just keep turning and everything turns. How does it feel to be part of the whole?"

"When I look at just me turning, it seems so simple, it seems easy. But I can get caught up in the whole, and when I see my importance in keeping everything going, it can feel overwhelming."

"But it is your job to just keep turning. Everyone else has their turning to do. You turn them but are not responsible for how they turn. If you can stop worrying about them turning and just turn yourself, that makes life so much easier. You are just turning, doing your job."

This dream demonstrated Raymond's ability to delegate and not take responsibility for everyone's work. He immortalized himself as just one gear. He salvaged an old gear from some abandoned equipment and began using it as a paperweight on his desk. His new found freedom, at least at work and in talking about his feelings with his wife, seemed to have become an unconscious part of him.

HROTHGAR ARRIVES

As Hrothgar stands on the threshold of Heorot, he praises this miracle of God, a miracle that no normal human could accomplish. He takes Beowulf as his own son and enters the blood-soaked hall; yet Heorot still stands. In response, Beowulf retorts that he regrets his failure to claim the life of Grendel, not that he didn't try his best, but God's will was to the contrary; Grendel would leave with his life, though mortally wounded, to suffer the eventual final judgement of God for his sins. Unferth, the orator of Hrothgar, notes that the talons of Grendel were made of steel, impossible to sever with a sword.

Finally, we consciously realize the overwhelming significance of our victory and how it has changed us. Our wise self, the king within, is conscious of the new strength now incorporated within us as the king takes Beowulf as a son. We also become conscious of the destroyed part of us, destroyed in the bloody battle. We remain standing, stronger than ever. We are not certain of the demise of our tormentor but know it suffered such a wound that it does not have the ability to harm us again. In addition, we now understand why our usual defenses were ineffective against the steel claws of our tormentor. The significance of what we have done becomes a conscious part of our wisdom, our wise self, the king within.

Megan felt victorious. She had felt empty, living in a void, lacking love. She had now learned to fill her emptiness with the love she was finding in the little things in life. Her dreams of the pool party at a friend's and her husband riding in a parade showed her that love was all around her. Her Christmas experience was full of love. People at work did appreciate her. Megan's new wisdom, the king within, had accepted her growing self-confidence and pride as a fact—pride in her work and in what she had to offer her husband. The king within has accepted her as a daughter. With confidence and pride her tormentor of depression has been rendered incapable of harming her.

Craig's emotional response to the hypnotic recall of his father's fight with Keith was a strong indication that some change had taken place within Craig. Talking about such an experience at the time of the experience can diminishes its effect. Talk tends to intellectualize the experience, diminishing its effect on the unconscious mind. Three weeks after the session seemed a better time for the King to return, for Craig to use the wise and benevolent part of himself to better understand what had happened.

Craig now could identify the qualities of love he and Keith needed from his parents: understanding, sympathy and patience—the qualities Craig's adult self had offered his younger self.

"Sit back and relax. Close your eyes. Breathe in calmness and, as you exhale, let that calmness go deeper inside you. Let yourself go back to the session of three weeks ago. You are sitting in your room. Your father has been yelling at Keith in the room next door. He now has stomped out. Your mother goes into Keith's room and she talks quietly. Then you hear her say 'Why can't you be more like Craig?' Your adult self goes back to help your younger self understand and to show your younger self love. Experience your adult self being with your younger self. What is happening?"

"I don't know. Nothing. He just puts his arm around me but says nothing."

"How does your adult self feel?"

"Very sad. I guess there is nothing for him to say."

"Your adult self just understands how scared and tied up your younger self feels. He needs to say nothing, but to just understand."

"He's holding me and that feels good."

"Tell me more about how that feels."

"When he held me I didn't feel scared, maybe just sad."

"Your adult self is sympathetic and understanding. In his quietness, in his willingness not to talk, you can feel his patience."

"Uh huh."

"Your adult self is understanding, patient, and sympathetic. Let those feelings grow within you. As an adult you have learned you can be understanding, patient and sympathetic in ways your parents didn't know."

Neither Craig's father nor his mother was able to be understanding, sympathetic, and patient. His father was critical and controlling and his mother was afraid. Because of her fear and her need to keep the peace, she seemed to lack patience and sympathy. The wise part of Craig has learned these feelings. The king within has brought Craig the gift of greater understanding.

The same words may be repeated many times, but just one time the listener may hear it differently. Sally looked at the print she and Bart had purchased of a woman dressed in blue sitting seductively in front of a mirror with her arms wrapped around one knee. Sally found meaning in the way the woman could admire and feel comfortable with herself. Though she had thought this many times, this time it struck her with a new understanding because she thought it about herself: "It is not being seductive to admire and feel comfortable with myself, and if I can admire myself why shouldn't Bart?" The wise king inside arrived with new understanding.

THE CELEBRATION GIFTS

Heorot is decorated for the great banquet. Beowulf enters and, after a toast in his honor, Hrothgar offers many magnificent gifts: an embroidered banner of gold, a helmet, a corselet, a jewel-studded sword. In addition, Beowulf receives eight horses with golden bridles and the king's own war saddle inlaid with jewels.

Our wise self, the king within, honors the warrior within, placing our warrior in front of all other warriors as banner carrier, with accouterments of the greatest warrior. We now appreciate and consciously realize our newfound exceptional male strength, the strength to take charge of our lives in a positive, assertive manner.

Craig felt reassured of his victory. He accepted his new strength of understanding, patience, and sympathy. Along with these female qualities, he felt new strength in his male qualities of the king: a new level of self confidence at work, and a new sense of self-confidence when meeting with his supervisor.

Sally tried sitting on the floor in front of the mirror on her closet door to admire herself. She had to get up to change from her slacks to a skirt but after sitting there for a few minutes the feeling of appreciation became part of her own self image. As Daniel Aaroz (1985) so well said, "It is not will power that produces change but imagination." Sally went beyond the use of will power to the use of her own image in the process of change.

During the next session with Sally and Bart, the week after their celebration party, I suggested we examine the changes in Sally. "Imagine the two Sallys, the old one sitting there and the new one over there. The old Sally feels out of control, vulnerable. The new Sally feels strong.

"The old Sally feels angry and afraid. What are some other words to describe the new Sally?"

"Not afraid or angry but, I guess, content, comfortable, maybe more adventurous or carefree, self confident."

"Does the word 'humiliated' describe the old Sally?"

"Uh huh."
"What does the new Sally feel?"
"Attractive, strong."

These words—strong, able to care for herself, adventurous, carefree, self-confident—describe the gift of the king, gifts of strength and assertiveness. As we shall see when the Queen Wealhtheow arrives in the story, the gifts of feeling attractive, content, comfortable are the gifts of the Queen, the gifts of receptivity, nurturance and warmth. With gifts from both the king and the queen, Sally finds greater balance in her life between her female and male sides.

Raymond was delegating responsibility at work and the results were good. He was the small wheel that got much moving. At home he shared his problems with his wife and she was empathetic. These changes were synergistic. The pressure of his problems at work were not so overwhelming, making it much easier for his wife to be empathetic rather than panic because he was panicking. As they shared his life, it became easier. The gift to Raymond was this realization.

A BALLAD IS SUNG

Songs are sung and ballads told as the banquet continues. One is the ballad of Hnaef a Danish warrior; Hildeburh, his sister; and the Frisian King Finn, the husband of Hildeburh. A quarrel occurred between the Danes and the Frisians. In this battle many were killed, including both Hnaef and Hildeburh's son. Hnaef's second in command, Hengst, then took charge of the battle. Both sides were so weakened that the small remaining band of Frisian warriors could not kill Hengst. Peace was made, and Finn offered to treat the remaining Danes honorably with gifts of victory equal to those of his own warriors. A funeral pyre was set for the Danish hero, Hnaef, and the grieving Hildeburh set her son on the pyre next to her brother.

Though unhappy, Hengst remained in Friesland for the winter. Finally, when offered a sword, he slew Finn in a surprise attack and returned to Denmark in honor with Hildeburh and the royal treasures of Finn.

This story of grief and honor, of death within a family, provides a metaphor for engraving in the unconscious the grief of loss of our old self and the respect and honor of our new self. Death is required for rebirth. Such death and rebirth stories of ancient times, as well as dreams, metaphor, and hypnotic experiences, access and change our unconscious mind. As we have seen, real change within us does not occur until it is registered within the unconscious mind. Telling ourselves consciously that we are strong or secure is not sufficient. We have to believe such characteristics unconsciously for them to become real within us. The grief and honor we have experienced in this process of therapy is engraved in our unconscious mind through stories. Stories remain with us after we have listened to them and they are available to our unconscious mind when our unconscious mind is ready to hear them.

To Sally, the death of her old self—the death of her vulnerability, weakness, humiliation, fear, and anger—seemed nothing over which to grieve. But this death required that Sally relinquish some features some women value: her soft, weak, vulnerable side. These female or receptive features found better balance with the growth in her assertive (male) side, her strength and self-confidence. Yet the female, receptive features of self-admiration and comfort grew.

I felt it was important for Raymond to have something more concrete at home as a reminder of his new realizations, like the gear on his desk at work was a reminder. But as we talked it became apparent that Raymond and his wife had already found this reminder in a ritual. Positive family rituals are important; though negative rituals can be destructive, positive rituals can insure the healthiness of a relationship. When Raymond got home from work, he and his wife would withdraw to Raymond's study. The study was the first place Raymond would go to drop his briefcase. His wife began following him there at first because of her concern. Now it had become a time just to spend a few minutes together to share the day. This ritual had become a beautiful and loving routine of homecoming, one that also reflects Wealhtheow's nurturance, as we shall soon see.

Aaron came for one more session. He truly felt victorious. I no longer could offer him a regular dose of skepticism. I had to join him in the victory parade, but I offered him one final hypnotic monologue and assignment. "You have given up a big piece of your life, the irresponsibility of your extramarital affairs. You feel great about your success in winning the confidence of your wife. You have given up the excitement and unconditionality of extramarital sex, and have won the confidence of your wife. You have not outwardly shown grief for your loss, the loss of the excitement and unconditionality of extramarital sex. You need to grieve and lay that irresponsible part of you to rest. Go out and find an urn. Write on a slip of paper your thoughts about the death of your extramarital affairs. Burn the note and place the ashes in the urn and place the urn in a prominent place for you to see as a continued reminder. Then, go for a walk through town with your wife, holding her hand in celebration of your new love. Renew your commitment at least once a month by going out together and walking through your community holding hands. Don't forget what has died while you appreciate your new life."

I told Peggy a brief metaphoric story. "You have taken this journey into the unknown with curiosity. You have been very strong, unusually strong. Many people have a much greater struggle on such journeys. It is painful for them to give up certain things in their lives. You easily gave up the wall of forgetfulness you built around a painful incident in your life. Many people would have shown greater fear or grief in giving up this wall. You did it with surprising ease. You looked at a painful time in your life and seemed to quickly resolve your fear or anxiety about it. There still may be other issues for you to deal with in the future, but for the time being, you found success. I'm here if you should want to talk with me in the future."

The ease with which Peggy faced the issue of playing doctor with Mike and Mike's mother opening the door, suggested to me that she continued to dissociate from that or other painful issues. I assumed she would soon return to therapy, but I felt she deserved support for what she felt was a significant victory. She had earned her victory banquet.

WEALHTHEOW ARRIVES

Queen Wealhtheow arrives at the banquet with her offerings to our hero. She presents Beowulf with an armlet, ring, and necklace. The necklace is comparable to the most beautiful Brosings' necklace of the Norse Goddess Freyja. She also honors him by asking him to be her sons' mentor.

The gifts of the King define Beowulf's masculinity. The gifts of the Queen strengthen his female aspects, offering him completeness and balance. She offers Beowulf beautiful jewelry symbolic of her female characteristics of attractiveness, sensitivity and soft sensuousness, symbolic of her receptive aspects of nurturing, healing, protecting, and loving others. This femaleness gives him balance with his hard male assertiveness or "insertiveness."

Moore and Gilette (1990) offer four main male archetypes: King, Warrior, Magician and Lover. I've suggested that the four female counterparts to these archetypes are the Nurturing Mother, Protective Mother, Healing Mother, and Sensuous Woman. These female archetypes are receptive rather than assertive, bringing others to them. Whereas the king provides outwardly for his people, the nurturing mother brings others to her breast. Whereas the warrior reaches out to attain some great accomplishment, the protective mother brings her people under her wing. Whereas the magician heals outwardly, the healing mother again brings others to her own body to heal—"I'll kiss it to make it well." Whereas the male lover experiences life with a passion and offers gifts of love, the sensuous woman brings others to her softness and love. The Queen's gifts offer Beowulf these receptive feminine qualities, providing him balance for his maleness.

Within us, this new found receptivity may take the form of greater intuition, sensitivity, patience, and softness in relating to others.

Though Craig gained a sense of self confidence in meeting with his boss, his other new attributes, his patience, sympathy, and understanding, were soft attributes offered him by the Queen.

Walking through his community holding hands with his wife was a continued reaffirmation for Aaron in his commitment to monogamy. This act said to the people he knew that he was committed and responsible. Both Aaron's male side and female side had been weak. He lacked assertiveness and the ability to take charge of his own behavior, but he also lacked an ability to receive love, to feel loved by others. With growing integrity, he felt more lovable and was more able to receive love, thereby strengthening his female, receptive side. His gift from the Queen was this ability to feel loved and appreciated.

Megan, too, had become more able to accept the love offered her. She had received the gift of greater receptivity from the Queen. Though she felt her job was a dead end, she now knew why she was not depressed when she went to work. She was appreciated there in numerous little ways. The thank yous and the smiles of others were small but important signs of appreciation. To the last hypnotic love strengthening exercise, I added, "As you inhale, be sensitive to what you inhale. Listen for the pleasant words from others and the pleasant smiles from others. Inhale those words and smiles. Appreciate these simple gifts you receive from others. Inhale those simple gifts. As you exhale, feel those gifts throughout your body. Receive them deeply within you."

Raymond's gift from the king was his ability to become more efficient and effective in dealing with problems in life without feeling overwhelmed by responsibility. His gift from the queen was his ability to be a better listener, receptive of other people's feelings, again without taking on the responsibility for their feelings. A time each evening was set aside in Raymond's study for this gift of nurturance.

FLUSHED WITH WINE

The celebration continues. Spirits are high and the troops become flushed with wine. They are unaware of what is in store for them. When night falls the King retires to his quarters. The benches are cleared away and bedding spread on the floor. The King's and Beowulf's men fall asleep in the great hall. At their heads lay their shields, and on the benches above them lay their helmets, corselets and spears.

We are confident our tormentor is dead. We lower our defenses and sleep soundly. We do not expect Grendel to return.

Megan had come a long way on her journey. Her spirits were greatly uplifted when she could accept the simple gifts of love from all around her. As her confidence grew in her sense of well being, she let go of her defenses. She wasn't as likely to think of possible ulterior motives when others thanked her or were pleasant to her. She let down her guard and was much more receptive and accepting.

For Sally the bedroom scene of getting dressed and undressed seemed very natural. She could look up and see Bart watching her. She could easily smile and he could smile too. Everything was feeling great.

Craig felt confident too. At the end of our last session I offered another hypnotic exercise. After trance induction, I suggested, "You are walking along a path through fields of wild flowers and wildlife. You are feeling good, feeling the fresh air of spring. As you walk through this meadow, ahead you see a stand of trees. You continue walking toward these trees, looking forward to sitting in their shade for a few minutes. As you approach the trees you see a tree stump that is an inviting seat. You walk to it, sit down and relax, enjoying the fresh air and beauty of spring. As you sit, you notice a very large tree nearby. As you inspect the bark of the tree, you notice a button on the tree, the kind of button you can push. You are curious and wondering, curious and wondering as you carry your thoughts of your experience of three weeks ago with you."

The experience three weeks ago had led Craig to define three needs: the needs for understanding, patience, and sympathy from his parents. I did not mention the needs in this induction because I wanted him to use his own perception of the importance of that session. Continuing, "You get up and push that button. To your surprise a door opens in the tree and you notice the inside looks like an elevator cab. You step in and notice above the door a row of numbers, numbers numbering downwards. Next to the door is a panel of buttons. At the top is 'G' for the ground floor. The buttons are numbered downwards, 1, down to 2, 3, on down to 10, down to 20, 40, down deeper 80, 100, deeper and deeper. Reach out and push one of the buttons. . . . The number in that button lights up. Read that number to me."

"Nine."

"The door closes and you feel the elevator begin to go down. The G light goes off and the one light goes on. . . . The 1 light goes off and the 2 light goes on. Down and down, curious and wondering as you take your thoughts of three weeks ago with you. The 5 light goes off as the 6 light goes on. Deeper and deeper. The 7 light goes off as the 8 light goes on. The 8 light goes off as you feel the elevator slowing down and the 9 light goes on. As the doors open, take a few moments for your eyes to adjust to see what is outside the door. . . . Take your time, go ahead and tell me what you see."

"It's beautiful, like the meadow I was walking in a few minutes ago. The flowers, the butterflies. It's so peaceful and the air is so fresh."

"Just stand there and enjoy what you see. When you are ready you can again push 'G' and let yourself really relax as you come back up and back to this office . . . . When you are ready you can open your eyes."

We decided this session would be the last, at least, for the time being, with the understanding that Craig could call me should the need occur. Craig seemed quite satisfied and felt that a number of issues in his life had been resolved. He had let down his defenses and assumed Grendel had been beaten. Like Megan, he was now flushed with wine.

CHAPTER VIII

Grendel's Mother

To this point in therapy the client has grown in emotional strength by facing and overcoming an immediate tormentor, one that came more or less unexpectedly into the life of the client. With this newly found emotional strength, the client is prepared to pursue the deeper source of his or her problem. After a short reprieve from torment with the celebration of the death of Grendel, from the unconscious mind arises an awareness of the deeper problem—Grendel's Mother. As the story of Grendel's Mother develops in this chapter, the first step for the therapist will be to "join" the client's fear and anxiety, helping the client define the nature of the problem—Hrothgar is Broken Hearted. The second step, "ego strengthening," will be to call upon the new found strength within the client—Beowulf Learns of the Night. Third, the client will need to accept the value and challenge of pursuing or uncovering the traumatic situation(s) or patterns from childhood—Beowulf Accepts the Challenge. Fourth, using the affect bridge, hypnotic regression will be used in the process of uncovering—Following the Blood of Aeschere. Fifth, as the client approaches the trauma, resistance will be experienced—Arriving at the Lake. Sixth, resistance will be overcome by renewing the clients focus on "intent, gentleness, and curiosity"—Beowulf's Preparation to Dive. These steps in the story of Grendel's Mother offers us, in greater detail, the elements necessary for using hypnotic regress to take a person hypnotically back through time.

GRENDEL'S MOTHER

Flushed with wine, the men bed down and fall asleep: the King in his quarters, Beowulf and his men in quarters assigned them in special consideration by the King, and the other men of the King in the great banquet hall.

Out in the moors broods Grendel's mother, grieving the loss of her son. Because Cain had killed his brother, he was banished by God to became an outlaw and made to relinquish human happiness to live in the wilderness. Likewise, Grendel's mother, banished by God, lives at the bottom of a murky lake. She, sad of heart because God had given Beowulf the wonderful gift of strength to kill her son, resolves to avenge her son's death.

We have relinquished our defenses, feeling satisfied with our victory over our tormentor. But we have yet to consider or face the genesis of our despair, Grendel's mother. We long ago dissociated ourselves from the abuse and trauma of our early years, from the feelings of abandonment as experienced by Scyld Scefing. We have gained great strength by overcoming our Grendel, and we are now ready to face Grendel's mother, to lower even further our defense of dissociation and face those early traumas. When we are most vulnerable, asleep, flushed with wine, the pain of this she-devil seeks expression. Her brooding sadness comes alive within us and begins to trouble us.

All six clients had reached a stage in therapy where they felt satisfied. They felt they had resolved a major problem in their lives, if not the only problem in their lives. Three had ended therapy; the others continued in therapy from once every two weeks to once a month. Each would experience the return of the old problem or an apparently new problem and return to a new round of intense therapy.

During the final session of therapy with Sally, the focus had been on her success in resolving her disgust with Bart watching her dress. Sally could dress in front of Bart feeling attractive and content. As usual, I suggest that if she felt a need she could telephone me in the future. One comment was made during the session that slipped by because of the excitement of the victory. Sally had mentioned that she and Bart had not had time for sex for several weeks. Grendel's mother was making herself known.

Craig had ended therapy but returned about eight months later. His obsessive worry about work had returned. Before he had been afraid of "gumming up the works." This time his fear was of having made a mistake or mistakes in his work, mistakes that had not yet been discovered. His fear and anxiety were as debilitating as ever.

Megan continued in therapy. I had been seeing her once every two weeks. Though I suggested we could end therapy, she stated that she felt a need to continue. Even though she was feeling good, she felt apprehensive. Her feelings were not stable. Often people who are depressed feel guilty about continuing in therapy, but Megan was not one of them. I trusted her intuition that something else was out there in the moor, that her apprehension had a legitimate basis. Her apprehension was focused on her parents' visit in a couple of weeks. Two days before they arrived, Megan phoned me for an appointment. I was able to see her the next day.

Megan was dreading the visit. She had been doing well, but she felt her parents would end all that. She didn't know why, except that she could "hear them bickering" and hated it. She had had difficulty sleeping for the last two nights, and she felt so sleepy at work that she occasionally dozed off for a few moments. Megan could feel the approach of Grendel's mother.

Aaron had been successful, and proud of his success, in being strong and protective of his family. He felt self-scorn when he thought seductively or fantasized when he saw one of his old girlfriends. The "mangy mutt" part of him was shrinking. Then, about six months after we had ended therapy, Aaron went to a week-long out-of-town training program for his work. While there, he met a woman with whom he ended up sleeping. On the way home he felt considerable disgust with himself, but he had the intent and commitment to not see the woman again. Though he felt mangy, Aaron believed he had sufficient control of himself to resist further temptation and did not consider resuming therapy. He was sure there would be no problem.

GRENDEL'S MOTHER ENTERS HEOROT

Grendel's mother bursts into the banquet hall onto the sleeping Danes. Because she is a female, she appears to these men to be of lesser strength than her son, no match for men armed with the sharpest hand-forged swords, swords that can pierce and bloody boar-armored helmets. The men snatch their swords and shields from above their heads, not thinking to grab their helmets or corselets.

As Grendel's mother first makes her presence known within us, we do not believe she can be strong enough to overcome our great strength. Our confidence now is such that we believe our weapons can defeat her. But the only weapons available at this unexpected moment are our old and usual defenses. Our new strength is asleep elsewhere.

One morning I went out to get the newspaper as usual and as I walked back to the house, I read the front page headlines. One article was about a local manufacturing plant downsizing. Raymond's name was in the second paragraph, and I wondered how he was doing. It didn't take long for me to find out. When I got to the office there was a message on the answering service for me to call him. Grendel's mother was on her way in.

Megan's folks arrived and she phoned me the next day. They had arrived that evening and the four of them had gone out to dinner. After returning home from dinner, her parents expressed a need to go to bed because they were tired after their trip. Their going to bed was no problem, actually a relief to Megan, until they closed the door to the guest bedroom. She could hear them begin to argue about the tip Megan's father had left the waitress and about the quality of the service. Megan wanted to scream, to barge into their room and tell them to leave if they could not get along without a fight. But she didn't—she ran to her bedroom, put the pillow over her head and tried to ignore the argument. Grendel's mother wreaked havoc within Megan.

Peggy had ended therapy feeling confident that her problems were solved. Peggy thought her "playing doctor" memory was no big deal, yet the amber lighting of the room seemed to match the flashes of an amber lit room she would see in her nightmares.

Several months had passed before Peggy called for another therapy appointment. Russ, her boyfriend, complained to her that she was again having night terrors and suggested she should again seek help. Her first thought was that the night terrors were no big deal. But to humor Russ, she came back to therapy.

Peggy's usual defense was dissociation. Though Grendel's mother had entered Hrothgar's banquet hall, she thought, "no big deal." This beast didn't appear as strong as Grendel, and to Peggy, even Grendel was a weakling, too. But Russ was more concerned, and Peggy realized she was again starting slowly in the morning, feeling tired and irritable. For a few weeks she had felt rested in the morning. Now the tired feeling had come back. She thought, "Maybe the therapist was right, there was more to my problem than the incident with Mike."

About two weeks went by after Aaron returned home from the conference; then he received an e-mail. The woman with whom he had slept at the conference reached out to him and he could not say no. The relationship resumed in cyberspace. They started having cybersex.

Grendel's mother came into the great hall. Aaron at first underestimated her strength—convincing himself that this was not a real affair, that cybersex was no problem. But one Saturday, his friend decided she had to talk with him and telephoned him at home. Sandy answered the phone.

GRENDEL'S MOTHER SEIZES AESCHERE AND RUNS

Grendel's mother hurries to seize one man from those sleeping in Heorot and makes a hasty retreat to her fens and lake. She takes Aeschere, Hrothgar's most loved counsellor and chieftain. She also retrieves the talon of her son while the men, seized in panic, fall into a state of gloom.

Grendel's mother has come unexpectedly and we are not ready with our new defenses. She comes and leaves quickly, leaving us in a state of panic and depression.

The morning before she made her appointment to see me, Peggy woke up in a sweat with a clear image of the amber lit room. She wasn't sure it was Jill's room. The lighting was amber but the room wasn't as nice or as neat as Jill's. She felt in a state of panic. Grendel's mother had grabbed one of Peggy's defenses, her dissociation or denial and run.

Aaron tried to convince his wife, Sandy, that this woman meant nothing to him, that he knew her only over the Internet, but this explanation did not satisfy her. Sandy's hope was destroyed. The more he tried to explain, the more he put his foot in his mouth, and the more upset his wife became. She couldn't believe he would try to justify a cyberaffair or think it meant nothing. Aaron just could not or would not understand Sandy's concern. Grendel's mother had run off with Aeschere. This crisis brought Aaron back to therapy.

Sally's progress in therapy had been significant. When Bart would look at her while she was dressing or undressing she could now feel appreciated, attractive, and comfortable. Sally knew that she could trust Bart and that he wasn't anything like the weird guy, Jake, who grabbed her in high school. We had felt confident in her victory and believed the problem was solved. Sally's rages at Bart had ended.

However, the problem was not resolved. Sally telephoned about six weeks later, quite upset. Bart was upset. She had lost interest in sex, she reported. Before, after her outbursts, Sally would feel guilty. She would make up to Bart by having dinner naked and having a "wild" evening. Now, Sally's need to make up had disappeared. She discovered that without the motivation of guilt, she had no interest in sex. She didn't mind dressing in front of Bart, but now she had no interest in exhibiting herself to him, either. Actually, she found herself avoiding exhibiting herself or dressing in front him because doing so might lead to sex. Needless to say, Bart was very upset. Grendel's mother had seized Aeschere and run.

Raymond had a great year, closer to two, before he returned to therapy. There was a crisis at work, a call from corporate headquarters to downsize. His neck and shoulder pain returned with a vengeance. He had no good way to delegate this responsibility of downsizing. Raymond had every right to be anxious, to be in pain. Though he tried to recall the relaxation exercises we had used and he still carried the yoked ox on his key chair, he could not find relief from this pain. The relaxation exercises lost their effect. He had become more irritable, though not explosive as before. Grendel's mother had wreaked revenge for the death of her son; the torment of Hrothgar returned.

HROTHGAR IS BROKEN HEARTED

Hrothgar is broken-hearted when he learns of the death of his most loved advisor. He immediately calls Beowulf to his chambers.

Our king within, the wise and benevolent part of ourselves, feels overwhelmed with despair upon the return of our tormentor. Yet, we do not feel the same sense of total hopelessness as before because we have our new strength to call upon. In therapy, the therapist, as a stand-in for the King, needs to offer the client understanding, joining the client in his or her feelings of hopeless and despair.

When Sally became aware of her lost interest in sex, and Bart helped make her aware of this loss, her king within was heartbroken. Then she was quick to call for help, seeking the understanding and reaffirmation of the therapist.

Raymond was disappointed in himself with the return of his pain. The king within was disappointed, broken-hearted. I reminded Raymond that each of us has our own way of experiencing stress. "Some of us get ulcers, others become so depressed they are unable to go to work. Some stop eating, some overeat. Though your way is painful, you continue to go to work. You are handling the downsizing situation as well as anyone could. That's why you were promoted to plant manager. If you didn't feel the pain in your neck and shoulders, you surely would have other problems, problems that could be worse. In any case, the time may be right for you to uncover when and how you learned your way. Better understanding your way of coping could improve your life. First, you learned that your neck and shoulder pain is caused by your need to please others and your fear of delegating responsibility. You then learned to delegate responsibility and trust others. By appreciating and trusting others, you allowed them to feel good about themselves. Yet, in this case, no one can appreciate the responsibility for having to downsize, for laying off employees. Before, you always had your father to go to. Now your parents live too far away. Your wife's a good listener, and, I'm sure, she is listening to a lot now, but there is no pleasant solution to this problem.

"Let's go on a journey to better understand why you store stress in your neck and shoulders."

Raymond was ready for the challenge of this journey, if for no other reason than to get his mind off his problem at work for just a few minutes.

It was time to join Craig in experiencing his emotional pain. His obsessive worry about work had returned. This time his worry was a little different. His work involved entering numbers and "number crunching" on the company's computer system. He was now afraid he had made a mistake or mistakes in dealing with these numbers.

As we may recall, Craig was a perfectionist, always seeking to please. He sought to please his critical and controlling father, which was impossible. His brother rebelled and didn't even try. His mother, trying to protect his brother from his father, would say, "Why can't you be more life Craig?" a statement Craig hated to hear, a statement that would tie him up in knots. He now realized how afraid his mother was of his father's anger. Over our first course of therapy, as this material surfaced, Craig's obsessive worry greatly diminished. He found greater self-confidence in talking to his boss, but now his obsessive worry had returned.

In "joining" Craig's emotional pain, my hypnotic monologue acknowledged, "You are very discouraged. Your worry has returned, as bad as ever. You just don't understand why you worry so. Every time you enter a number into the computer you check and recheck, but you still worry the number may have been wrong. It's getting so bad you are starting to get behind in your work. You are spending too much time checking and rechecking. You try so hard to do a good job and you are so afraid you will screw up. Your boss has started to show you greater respect when you tell him of your thoughts and feelings, but now you are afraid you can loose his respect if you make a mistake. You come home at night exhausted from all the worry. You feel things are hopeless. You thought you had your problems solved after uncovering those feelings you had when you were young, but that now seems to have not been the problem. There must be a deeper problem . . . ."

The "yes-set" had been established—Craig had been answering "yes" to himself to each of my statements. I could see his answer in a very slight nod of his head. He was looking down, but was in a trance. When someone else joined him in his emotional pain—his broken heart—the pain did not feel quite as overwhelming.

The next morning after her parents' argument, Megan left the house in anger before her parents were up. She was not willing to fix breakfast for them but left the task to her husband. Feeling hopeless in her emptiness, Megan was furious that her parents had done this to her. It was too early to phone me, and Megan had the day off work so she couldn't escape there, she ended up just driving around. She finally parked in a lot next to the park, just leaned back and thought. Her greatest resentment was how her parents could take away her feeling of happiness: "It is unfair. My parents should want me to be happy, should want the best for me, but instead all they do is cause me grief and pain. That's not the way life should be. I should feel safe and protected when I'm with them, not frightened and empty. It's so unfair." Megan was broken-hearted. She felt life was hopeless. I listened to this story that afternoon when I could first make time to see her.

BEOWULF LEARNS OF THE NIGHT

Beowulf arrives at daybreak and greets Hrothgar with pleasantries, not knowing of the demise of Aeschere. The tormented King tells of the terror of the night, of the monster killing his loved counsellor. He notes that the people of his kingdom and his counsellors have spoke not only of the one they call Grendel but also of another they recognize as female. Both are larger than human and live in a Godforsaken lake not too far from Heorot. Every night a terrible spectacle of fire is seen over the lake. It is so terrifying that even a deer cornered by hunters at the lake's edge will rather die than jump into the lake to escape. Hrothgar asks Beowulf for his help, believing only he can rid the country of this monster. He offers Beowulf great ancient treasures of gold if he succeeds.

The existence of this new tormentor within us was known, but only through rumors. We have sensed this tormentor, possibly through occasional dreams, but we wanted to deny its existence. But what we have ignored we now have to accept. Our defense of rationalization or denial is gone and we are forced to face reality. Our wise self now grieves and tells our warrior self the rest of what we know. In our grief, we begin to think through the situation and pull together our strength. We hear and accept the proclamations of our therapist, who is one voice of our wise king: our work is not finished. We have to face our tormentor with strength, curiosity and determination. Only then will we win.

My hypnotic monologue for Craig continued: "There must be something deeper. Something else is bothering you, and we can find it. You returned to therapy because you are ready to go after it and to find it. Even though you feel hopeless despair, you are now stronger than you were a year ago when you first came to therapy. You have learned a lot about yourself. Your new knowledge gives you the strength to dig deeper, to uncover more painful things in your life.

By the return of your worry, your unconscious mind is saying you are now ready, now strong enough, to take on these deeper issues."

With the establishment of the yes-set, my words become the words of Craig's wise self, his king within, and so the warrior within is called upon to take up the new challenge. With each statement, Craig is able to answer "yes."

Sally's lack of interest in sex suggests that there is more to her problem than dealing with the Jake issue. Sally recognized this herself: "I thought the Jake issue was finished. What more could there be?" Her question suggested that unconsciously she knew there was more to uncover and gave us direction for the next session.

Megan felt her life was hopeless. Her parent's fight and her inability to shut it out with her head under the pillow caused her to panic. She felt more depressed than ever. Megan hadn't considered herself depressed before therapy, but once she found that life could be happy and enjoyable, she realized that she had indeed been depressed. Yet the intensity of her reaction to her parents' fight suggested that there must be something deeper troubling her. Although at first her inner warrior had fallen asleep without a clue of a greater problem, Megan now began awakening to its existence.

We talked about what Megan had learned the first time around, about how she could come out of her depression. She pulled out of her purse the pin, "God Loves Simple Things," and put it on.

"You learned that happiness only happens in the moment. You have found happiness and peace in the simple things of life, the simple smiles of others and their thanks. Life was starting to become pleasant, but then your parents came and the pleasantness of the simple things flew out the window. All your old feelings and habits came rushing back.

"Take a few minutes to slow down and find peace in the moment. You are away from your parents for the moment. Take a moment to notice your breathing. Let your breathing slow down, let your breathing flow deep within you. With each breath inhale peace and calmness; with each breath, exhale, letting the peace and calmness go deeper within you. Feel yourself slowing down, feel the quiet and peace in this office. Feel yourself relaxing deeper and deeper. Appreciate the moment. When you leave here and walk the short distance back to work, feel the peace and calmness you have been experiencing at work. Appreciate the smiles and "thank yous" you get at work.

"Let the peace and calmness within you grow, and when you leave work to go home, prepare yourself to find and see the peace and calmness at home. You know there will be moments at home with your parents visiting when you will loose that peace and calmness. When you loose it, when your parents bicker, let their bickering be their problem, not your problem, let their bickering be their problem. When they bicker you can find something else simple and pleasant for your focus of attention to find peace and calmness. Relax and inhale a sense of peace and calmness."

The wise part of Megan was ready to accept the warrior, her ability to find peace and calmness, in her chambers. She had learned to call upon Beowulf, and she believed she could do it now. She accepted the challenge.

Aaron returned to therapy. He at first refused to admit that a cyberaffair was a problem, insisting it was not a "real" affair. He returned only because his wife insisted. I suggested, "Close your eyes, sit back and relax. Recall one of your old girl friends, the one you saw most recently. Sometimes after seeing one of your old girl friends, you would fantasize about her, fantasize being in a motel room with her, fantasize undressing her, fantasize having sex with her. Now, with the woman you met and communicated with over the Internet, you have sex. You masturbate while she writes you messages. You fantasize about her. You listen to her sexy talk and it excites you. You fantasize, yet you decided some time ago the fantasies you had about old girl friends were wrong and worthy of scorn. When you fantasized, you were being weak, not protective of your family. You were indulging in your need for unconditional but irresponsible love. You had no real love for these woman other than to fill your indulgent need. These fantasies became scornful to you. Now you are indulging in fantasies over the Internet. You are again fulfilling your indulgent need. Let the feeling of self-scorn return. You have a problem. We can track it down to its source, work to heal those wounds, find a way to change the way you look at the world.

"Sit there for a few moments. Feel the scornfulness grow, as you let your attention return to the present." Aaron was ready to admit he still had a problem. His acceptance of my words in trance indicated that he felt scornful of himself and was ready to take on the challenge.

BEOWULF ACCEPTS THE CHALLENGE

"We all must die, and a dead man's best memorial is the fame he wins before death." With these words, Beowulf states his allegiance to his friend and accepts the challenge to track and kill the mother of Grendel.

Even with a tormentor more frightening than death itself, we will win if we face it with strength, confidence, and curiosity. We have only one good choice. If we run it will chase us. If we hide it will find us. Our only choice is to stand up and face it. This time, rather than sit back and wait for it to come to us, with determination we pledge to go after it, track it down, and kill it.

Aaron accepted the challenge by deciding to not answer his cyberfriend's messages. To him that seemed easier than ending a real affair, but still he knew some deeper issue needed to be faced in therapy.

Megan also accepted the challenge. She left my office with every intent to find peace and calmness in the moment. But once she got home to her visiting parents, this task was easier said than done.

During our next session, Peggy was more serious than before. Earlier she had had a "no big deal" attitude. This time she looked more panicked. The amber lit room was not the room of her friend Jill. She now knew there was something deeper. To help Peggy's inner warrior accept the new challenge, I sought to help her renew her inner strength with the suggestions, "Recall your journey to this point, your journey toward the amber lit room. That room seems important, so central to your nightmares. The journey began with a vague feeling and moved toward greater clarity to the room of your friend, Jill. But the room in your dream was disheveled, Jill's was not. You wonder, you're curious. You've come a long way in your journey. You have found strength in your journey. Your nightmare of the amber lit room tells me you have sufficient strength, strength you have gained on this journey. You are ready to continue on this journey. Your unconscious mind is telling you that you are ready to move ahead to uncover some trauma in your life. Your dream says that your unconscious mind has accepted this challenge. So let's again begin the journey."

For Craig, too, there must be something more, for he was again stuck with his obsessive-compulsive fear. During our earlier course of therapy Craig went back through time to the cabin in the woods and later back to when his father stomped out of the house in anger at Keith. Craig was much stronger now than before and might be ready to face that deeper problem, but as a precaution to avoid a possible failure, I decided to proceed by looking for a clue to that deeper problem using another hypnotic technique.

"Think about sitting in front of your computer entering numbers and feel within you the sense of growing fear that makes you check and check again. Stay with that feeling and let it carry you along as you get up from your computer and walk to the elevator. Let that feeling carry you along as you get on the elevator and press the very bottom button on the elevator panel. Let that feeling carry you along as the elevator carries you down. This time it goes down and down to floors you have never been to, down and down to floors you did not know this elevator would go to. As you go down and down you are curious and wondering where it will take you knowing that where it is taking you will give you a clue about your fears. As it carries you down you watch the lights go on and off on the light panel above the door. You notice the lights are approaching the bottom floor and you are curious and wondering what you will find. Soon the elevator slows to a stop with a slight bump. When you feel that bump you know that the doors will soon open and you are curious and wondering about the nature of the clue.... Now you feel the bump and the doors open.... Take your time as you notice what is outside the door.... When you are ready to tell me what you see go ahead."

After a pause Craig slowly began: "It's a bright room with an old double bed. It smells musty. It seems familiar. It's small with a high ceiling but part of the ceiling slopes down. Pink flowered wall paper, old and cracked. Blue ceiling. I know I've been here before but I can't remember."

"How do you feel?"

"Hot, very hot, sweating. My heart is racing. I'm beginning to feel sick to my stomach."

"Okay. Is there anything else you want to do, or are you ready to go back up?"

"I'm ready to go back up."

"Okay. Look at the panel of elevator buttons. Pick the button of the floor for your office and push it. As the elevator goes up take a few deep breaths and let each breath relax your stomach. By the time you get to your floor your stomach will be relaxed and you will have cooled down. Take the image of that bedroom with you with patience, gentleness, and curiosity."

FOLLOWING THE BLOOD OF AESCHERE

Beowulf continues to speak. "She has no hiding place, whether in the bowels of the earth, in a mountain thicket or at the depths of the ocean, where I could not find her." Hrothgar and the warrior/prince set out royally on horses while their troops join them on foot. The path of blood is clearly visible on the ground, through the forest, over rocky ground, and on the forbidden paths of demons.

We begin our journey to track this monster, a journey into our unconscious mind of forgotten memories, a journey with pitfalls; but the path is clear. This journey takes us through dreams and hypnotic experiences to face the early traumas in our lives.

Again we used time regression, using the image of an amber lit room as the bridge. Peggy's journey had first taken her to her friend's room. However, Jill's room felt safe and comfortable. It was not the room of a traumatic experience. Now Peggy was tracking Grendel's mother to her lair.

Craig mentioned the image of the bedroom to his mother. She told him that it sounded sort of like a bedroom in the old farm house where his grandparents lived at one time. He did not remember that house, but he was on the trail of the blood.

Aaron demonstrated his readiness to track the blood of Aeschere to the lair of the fiend. He quickly went back through time to the time of his father's sermons condemning the evils of sex, but recalling these sermons were nothing new to him. He talked again about going to a Christian college and his sexual rebellion. He talked about his lack of interest in going to church. He had talked much about these earlier life experiences and feelings in earlier sessions of therapy, but we knew by his new level of high emotional energy that he was on the trail.

Sally was very ready to begin her renewed journey. I suggested that there must be something more in her personal history, something that was affecting her feelings about sex. Was it possible that the issues involving Jake had not been resolved, or was there something else that had happened? I was unwilling to rule out either.

I suggested we begin with time regression, using as a bridge her lack of interest in sex. She lifted her finger. "What is going on?"

"I'm at home talking with my mother."

"How old are you?"

"Oh, 16, it's the same day I was grabbed by that idiot."

"What's going on?"

"My mother asked me what I was doing. I told her I was just in the lunch line talking to a friend. I didn't even notice who was behind me. She told me that everything will be okay, but I think she thinks it was my fault."

"Let your adult self go back and be with your 16-year-old self. With all the wisdom and understanding of your adult self, help your younger self understand, help your younger self find the best words to describe how you feel."

"I was pissed off at her but didn't say anything."

"Go ahead."

"I was angry."

"Stay with your anger. Beneath that anger are more specific feelings, possibly hurt because she didn't trust you. You possibly felt humiliated . . . guilty . . . frustrated. . . . Feel your anger. Let your adult self help you find your more specific feelings."

"Hurt. She didn't trust me. Frustrated, because I couldn't get her to understand."

"So often people feel guilty even for things they didn't do, they feel they could have done something to stop it from happening. You are a person who quickly feels guilt in other situations."

"Maybe I feel a little guilty, but I don't think so. I didn't do anything wrong."

"Okay, recognize and feel your hurt and frustration. You mother didn't understand you and didn't trust you. Let those feelings become clear to you. . . .

"Now, again let your adult self go back and be with your younger self. Help your younger self find the best words to describe what you need. You need your mother to trust you and understand you. Help your younger self find more ways to say what you need. Talk to the mother image inside of you. Tell her what you need. 'Mother, I need you to trust me. Mother, I need you to understand how humiliated I felt when I was grabbed, when I was called into the principal's office.' Think of other ways you can say what you need."

"Mother, I need you to listen to me. Mother I need you to believe me." Sally sat quietly.

"Good. This week I want you to start a notebook, a journal. Write down all the words you can think of to describe how you felt and all things you need from your mother. Start with the ones we already mentioned. Now, take several breaths. With each breath let your attention gradually come back to the present."

Sally began the journey to uncover the source of her problem—she began tracking the blood of Aeschere.

Raymond too was eager to begin his journey. Even though he understood he had sufficient cause for the neck and shoulder pain, and that other physical ways of reacting to emotional stress could be as bad or worse, the pain was such that he wanted to find a solution. Also, the journey to understand the source of his pain could be at least a temporary distraction from its current cause, the corporate downsizing.

We began time regression using Raymond's neck and shoulder pain as the bridge. Raymond was quick to return to an incident we had examined before, the day before he began kindergarten. He and his mother had gone shopping for school clothes, and he was excited about starting school. That night he wet his bed and was very upset about it. He pulled the sheets off his bed and hid them in the closet. He was scared of what his father would think or do. He knew "big boys" didn't wet the bed.

When Raymond's mother came in to wake him the next morning, she was very sympathetic. She understood how excited he was about school and how he would not want her to tell his father. Raymond not only needed very much to please his dad but was also intimidated by and afraid of him. I suggested to Raymond, "Feel and hold onto your feelings of fear and anxiety about your daddy finding out about your accident. Let those feelings grow within you." I was preparing Raymond to take a different affect bridge further back in time, the bridge of his fear of his father. Raymond was tracking Grendel's mother to her den.

ARRIVING AT THE LAKE

Suddenly the men come to the bloodstained lake. There they are shocked to find the head of Aeschere on a rock overlooking the lake. Swarms of reptiles inhabit the water, strange dragons and monsters. As the horn for the troops blasts, the water monsters plunge deeper. With his bow, Beowulf kills one fierce water beast. They drag it onto the bluff to examine this ghastly creature.

As we reach the depths of our unconscious mind, we find the painful trauma of our early years—trauma that may be obvious, such as clear physical, sexual or emotional abuse, or subtle, such as destructive or limiting behaviors and attitudes or discipline. When we reach this lake of torment and abuse within our unconscious mind, we see in it the tormenting trauma and abuse, and we prepare to dive in and confront our tormentor directly.

I instructed Raymond, "Go back even further in time, this time carrying your worry or fear of your daddy with you."

Raymond found himself again with his mother. "I am standing next to my wagon and the wheel is off. Mommy is saying 'what will daddy say?' I feel like I'm going to cry."

"Again, let your wise and understanding adult self go back and be with your four-year-old self. Help your four-year-old self understand. What does he understand?"

"Daddy is going to be mad at me for breaking my wagon."

"Let you adult self help your younger self understand what you need from daddy."

"I need daddy to not be mean, to not punish me."

"Can you put that into a positive statement? What do you need?"

"I need daddy to be patient and to be gentle."

"Okay, when you say to yourself you need daddy to be patient and gentle, say that to the daddy inside of you, feel a sense of patience and gentleness grow within you as you deal with your family and people at work. Let this patience and gentleness grow within you. . . .

"Now, again, when you are ready, let yourself go back even further in time. Carry the feeling of fear or worry about your daddy back even further. Be patient and wondering as you go back further. When something catches your attention, lift the index finger of your right hand. . . ."

After some time Raymond spoke up saying that nothing was happening, nothing was coming to mind. The hour was close to being over so I suggested, "We can and will come back to this moment. Take your time, take several deep breaths, relax, feel patience and gentleness growing within you. . . . When you are ready you can again open your eyes."

Raymond was at the edge of the lake. Monsters could be imagined on the journey ahead. He needed some preparation to dive. I believed the dive was ahead of him because I had not seen a significant emotional release on the journey to this point. One question was beginning to form in my mind. Raymond had a lot of respect for his father and enjoyed sharing his life with him, even though at times his father might give him advice or a fatherly lecture. This advice or lecture annoyed Raymond because he felt his father should trust him more. Yet there was no evidence so far of his father abusing him, even though we were on a journey expecting to uncover such abuse. I began to suspect that his mother's pattern of planting suggestions that his father could "get mad" was more abusive than actual actions of his father. In either case, monsters could be seen in the murky waters ahead.

Sally came to the lake of resistance when she realized that her problem continued even as we were working through her feelings about Jake. She wrote regularly in her journal as I had suggested. The next time I saw her I added a journaling assignment. "As you address your inner mother, as you tell your inner mother what you need, the mother within will listen to you and work to become a better mother. Examine what you do each day in your relationships with others, with Bart and people with whom you work. Write down examples of how you are becoming a better mother in your relationships with others, how you meet the needs of others, the needs you needed met by your mother. Note how you better listen to others, better trust others, better understand others when they are hurt or humiliated. Write down how the mother within you is becoming healthier."

Sally felt good about the assignment. She knew there was something else to explore because her interest in sex actually diminished. The emotional pain she was causing her husband, and felt herself, encouraged her to go on. She needed to go deeper into her unconscious, and these journaling experiences were preparing her to dive into the lake.

When Megan got home that night it was not long before she was in her room crying. She could not stand her parents. She had the intent to face them with peace and calmness, and she was even gentle with herself in that she did not feel depressed about being depressed. She allowed herself the right to be frustrated and angry with her parents. But she had very little patience with them, and she forgot about being curious about the source of her feeling. She thought she knew where her frustration came from—she blamed them.

Though Megan went to bed crying, she woke in the morning with a dream that provided her with some relief.

"I was watching a dog and cat fighting. The dog was a big drooling kind of dog with a deep bark, not the kind of dog who would hurt anybody. The cat was hissing and swatting at the dog but the dog kept a good distance, kept backing away. The dog was just tormenting the cat. It was a stupid fight, a no brainer. Finally the dog got just a little too close and got scratched on the end of its nose. It went away with its tail between its legs. There was no purpose to the fight. They were fighting as if they knew they were supposed to fight but didn't know why. I woke relaxed thinking how stupid it was to fight, like my folk's fights are stupid."

I thought there was something more to the dream than did Megan. She found it gave her a new perspective and some freedom from her parent's bickering. Arriving at the lake was not as frightening for Megan as I might have expected. Something felt wrong to me.

The bedroom clue prepared Craig to again go back through time, hopeful that the clue would open the door to his earlier years. We used his obsessive worry as an affect bridge as he again began to go back through time. During this session, as he went back, being curious and wondering, Craig experienced more clearly a barrier to going back. He recalled his tenth birthday and how excited he was that his father had built him a go-cart that he could ride around in the fields behind their house.

"Okay, as you stand there, the day before your tenth birthday, look back through time, look into the past, tell me what you see. Take your time as you look back, what does it look like?"

"Nothing. I see nothing."

"Take your time. What does that nothing look like? When people see nothing, sometimes the nothing can take some form. Take your time. Does it have a color, or a temperature, or a sound?"

"Yeah. I see the color red, it's hot. Sound, I don't know. I hear a buzzing sound, like my ears are ringing."

"Look into the red. Is there any substance, or is it empty space?"

"I guess it's empty space. Some red seems further away than other red. It's more like sheets of light, or foggy light, like maybe red light shining on a thin cloth, what do you say, like cheese cloth or like curtain material. Some curtains are hanging or stretched from the top to the bottom, closer than other curtains. Some curtains are stretched horizontal too, with red light shining on them."

"Look through those curtains. Can you see anything?"

"No, except maybe shadows, but I can't make out what the shadows could be."

"Some curtains are further away than others. How many curtains do you see?"

"Oh, maybe four or five. One is only a few inches from me. The furthest one might be 20 feet away."

"Can you see beyond them?"

"No. Where they cross or when one is behind the other, it is dark red, but where there is only one layer of cloth, it is light red, but there are enough curtains that I can't see through or beyond them. The shadows seem to be between the layers of curtains."

"At first you said what you saw was hot. How is it hot?"

"I'm hot. I feel like I am sweating."

"Can you tell me more about the hotness? Like, where is it coming from or what is causing it?

"Those shadows I see. I feel sick to my stomach and hot, when I try to see those shadows."

"Okay, just stay there, look into the red curtains. Take a few deep, calming breaths, let yourself relax and cool down as you look into the pieces of red cloth. Be curious about the red curtains. It's important to keep looking into them and coming back to them until you can see what's behind them, between them. If you start to get too hot or anxious you can go back to your birthday party or your new go-cart, but know that you will come back to those curtains."

Craig was looking into the lake of Grendel's mother with its monsters, into the unknown of his past. Though he had yet to dive in, he could feel the apprehension and fear of facing the trauma of his childhood.

BEOWULF'S PREPARATION TO DIVE

These monsters do not dissuade Beowulf from donning his armor, his corselet, helmet, and the sword tempered in blood—all decorated with gold and jewels, the wonderful treasures of the king. The famous sword, lent him by Unferth, has never failed in battle. Before, Unferth had expressed jealous disdain for Beowulf, but now he has relinquished his reputation as hero, and his support is offered and appreciated.

Before the plunge, Beowulf asks that if he should die, Hrothgar stand in the place of a father for him, and that he look after his companions. He also asks the king to send the treasures given him to Hygelac, Beowulf's uncle and the king of the Geats, and to give Unferth his sword if Unferth's treasured sword should be lost.

Before we enter this world of tormenting family behaviors and attitudes, we need to prepare ourselves, to arm ourselves with strength and confidence, to stalk greater understanding with intent. We need to arm ourselves with the right attitude. This attitude seems best described with three words: intent, curiosity, and gentleness. We need to prepare ourselves with the *intent* to change our habits or life patterns. Such changes are not easy and, when we backslide or make mistakes, we need to be *gentle* with ourselves. Third, when we backslide, we need to examine what happened with *curiosity,* allowing this curiosity to help us understand and learn from our mistakes. Curiosity also opens our mind to the unknown, as we journey through the unconscious mind. These three words come from three very different traditions. The word intent is from the writings of Carlos Castaneda, used in his description of the process of seeking personal power. Gentleness is from the teaching of Transcendental Mediation: as one mediates and one's mind wanders, one gently brings attention back to one's mantra. Curiosity comes from hypnosis: "Be curious and wonder as you go back through time." It is a word to facilitate dissociation. Dissociation can lessen fear and make it bearable to proceed into the unknown. With this armament, we are ready to enter the lake of our torment.

We honor our wisdom, Hrothgar, who gives us the strength of *intent* to go on this journey, asking his wisdom to take care of us. We honor the healthy part of our past, our ancestry, Hygelac, accepting the fact that it is our ancestry that brought us to this point in life, giving us the self confidence and freedom to act. This part of us has received very little thought or appreciation during this journey, yet it looks on, not with fear and protective control, but with the freedom of loving *curiosity,* watching us as we journey into the unknown. And we honor even the weak, frightened, or dishonored part of ourselves, Unferth, recognizing this human side of us with *gentleness.*

Our previous self doubt, represented by Unferth, now has been transformed into respect for our commitment and strength and the knowledge that we have to move ahead, to plunge into this lake. Our formerly self-doubting, critical part now offers us a weapon to cut through the muck, a weapon that has never failed, a decisive weapon that allows us to discriminate between right and wrong, the real and unreal, on our journey into the lake. In turn, we know we have nothing to loose; even our life is less important than finding freedom from our torment. We accept the possibility of our death, making the necessary arrangement for it, which gives us an even greater sense of strength and freedom in facing our tormentor.

The hypnotic monologue with Craig resumed with the following ego strengthening words: "As you search through these walls of red lit curtains, as you search through your past, you will soon come upon those incidents in your early life that have affected you in your adult life, incidents that taught you your habits of fear and obsessive worry. You now have the strength and are ready to face the torment of your past. As you venture into your past with the intent to uncover these incidents, you are curious and wondering, curious and wondering about what you will find. Your adult self is strong and gentle. Your adult self knows how to relate to your younger self with gentle patience. As you venture into your past, you will find those incidents, those patterns of your childhood that caused you torment. Your adult self will need to care for your younger self with gentle patience to help him understand and deal with the torment. You are prepared to find what is behind those red lit curtains, to find what happened before you were ten years old. Be gentle and curious as you journey into your past."

As the session with Megan continued, I suggested, "You know how your parents are and you have these expectations of them. With this understanding and with some patience you can overcome your frustration, but there may be other things that have happened between you and your parents that are keeping your frustration alive. Let's track them down. Take a few deep breaths, relax, and let yourself go into a trance. You have become very good at going into a trance. Good. Again, carry your feelings of frustration with you. Curious and wondering, let yourself go back in time. Go back to a time before the time you were sitting in the dark closet. Go way back. Watch your life go by and soon something will catch your attention."

Without me even asking, she lifted her finger. "Again I'm in darkness . . ."

"What's that darkness like?"

"It's thick. It's like I'm in warm black water."

"What's happening? What are you doing?"

"Nothing. I'm just there."

"Standing? Sitting?"

"I don't know. It's not like I have a body. I'm just there."

"Okay, just be there. Relax, be curious. Take your time and see what happens."

We sat for about ten minutes. I occasionally suggested: "Relax, be curious. Take your time and see what happens." But Megan had to get back to work, so I concluded the session, "Remember where you are. Take this experience with you with curiosity and wonder. We will come back to it. Now, follow for a few moments your breathing. With each breath let yourself gently relax with curiosity and wonder. When you are ready you can open your eyes and let your attention come back to this office."

Megan had reached a barrier in her journey into her unconscious. She was at the lake's edge, preparing herself to dive in. She was prepared with intent, curiosity, and gentleness. She did not show anxiety or fear about the experience of blackness and was ready to return to it the next session.

During Aaron's next session he mentioned he really wanted to be the loving protector of the family, the German Shepherd, but he did not understand what gets in the way.

I suggested that we look at Aaron's two parts more carefully—one, the mangy mutt, and two, the German Shepherd. Pointing to one chair, I suggested, "There sits the mangy mutt" and to another chair, "there sits the German Shepherd. Using Aaron's earlier descriptors I indicated "The mangy mutt is dirty, disgusting, a stray, just wanders around. Yet he can be very loyal. There the German Shepherd is strong, reliable, the protector, loving, and faithful. Let those dogs become parts of you in those chairs and tell me what you see."

Indicating the mutt chair, Aaron said, "I feel like a stray, that I don't belong. I guess that's the way I have always felt. The Shepherd, I don't know. I've never felt strong or reliable, but always uncomfortable and itchy." The German Shepherd seemed totally foreign to him. His thoughts were preparatory, opening the door for the next session.

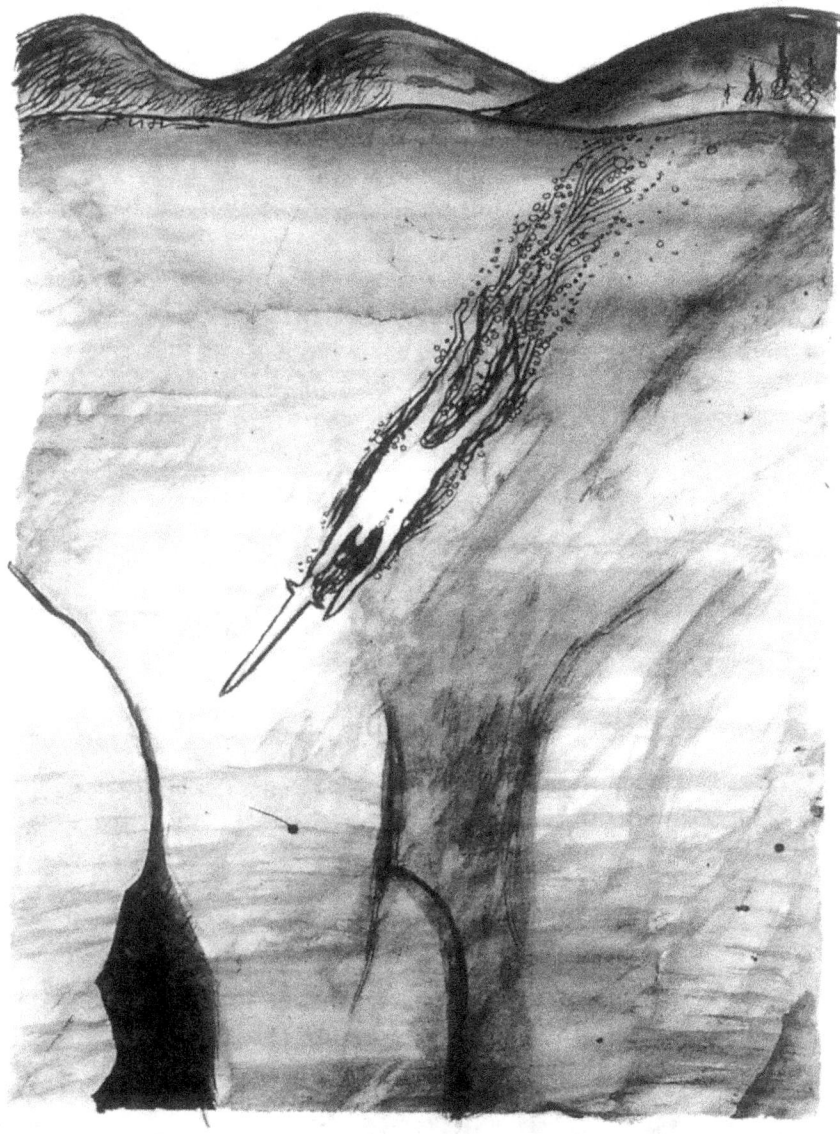

148 / GRENDEL AND HIS MOTHER

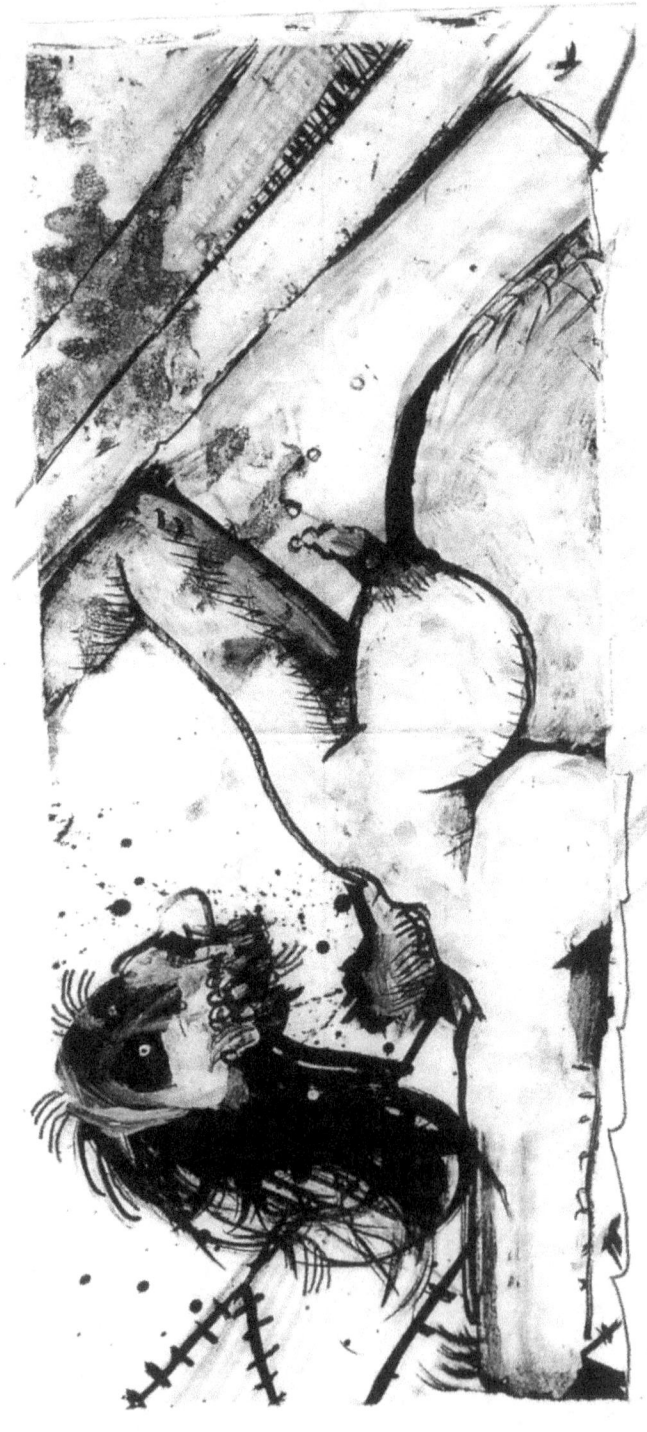

CHAPTER IX

The Death of Grendel's Mother

GETTING TO THE BOTTOM

Beowulf sets off for the bottom of the lake, plunging into the water. He takes the better part of a day to reach the bottom. We now venture into the untouched reaches of our unconscious mind, those unknown areas into which we have never in our conscious memory ventured. This destination frequently requires going into a deeper trance than before and/or finding new ways around fear and unconscious resistance. This territory may be unknown verbally because it may have been first experienced during the pre-verbal phase of our life, those early years when we did not have the language ability to express our feelings or needs; or it may be unknown because of the defense of dissociation from the severe pain, emotional or physical, of an ancient incident. At a deep emotional level, however, we know the destination.

During our last session Megan was floating in thick darkness—black water. During the next session, I told her we could now return to this experience. She was ready to dive in. As we continued this hypnotic experience, the water became thicker and warmer. Megan felt herself suffocating. She found herself lying in her bed in a state of panic. Again she could hear her parents fighting downstairs. She pulled the covers over her head and put her head under the pillow, terrified, wanting them to end the fight. In the therapy session, she was breathing hard, close to hyper-ventilating. Tears and sweat were running down her cheek. She was terrified by the fight. We knew we were close to something important.

Peggy had returned to therapy because of the return of her nightmares and the recurring recollection of the amber lit room. She was very ready to plunge into the dark recesses of her unconscious mind. As she went into a trance, Peggy quickly regressed to about the age of three, lying in her crib for her afternoon nap. The amber color was of her room with the shades closed. There was nothing frightening about that experience; in fact, it was pleasant and warm. Her mother was reading her a story before she fell asleep.

I suggested she go back even further in time.

"There is nothing."

"You are experiencing nothing. What is that like? Take some time to examine it. . . . What is it like? Is it light or dark?"

"It's dark with splotches of white or light."

"Go ahead. What do you feel?"

"I'm warm. I don't see anything. Just black with splotches of light. I feel very light, like I am floating."

"Just stay with that feeling and see where it takes you. Be curious and wondering as you float through the dark with splotches of light. Take your time. Be curious to see where it takes you."

After about ten minutes, with occasional prompting about curiosity and wondering, floating, dark with splotches of light, and "seeing where it takes you," Peggy eventually began to see more light, amber light, an amber lit bedroom, with the bedding a mess on the bed.

Peggy was at the bottom of the lake. The sea hag was carrying her to her den.

The next session with Aaron began with using the mangy mutt as the bridge back through time. While he was in trance I asked him to describe the mangy mutt.

"Its fur is dirty and disgusting. I wouldn't want to touch it. When I look at it, it makes me itch all over. There are places where the skin is bare, it's red and oozing. The fur is scabby and oily. It's slimy. It's disgusting."

"Okay, feel yourself itching all over with red oozing skin, scabby, oily and slimy, as you go back through time. Be curious and wondering as your life goes by, year by year, people, places, seasons, feeling yourself covered with mange . . ."

After a few minutes Aaron lifted his finger.

"Okay, what's happening?"

"My father just came home. He is just standing there looking at me with his look of scorn."

"How old are you? What's going on?"

"I guess I'm about 12 years old. He's just looking at me with his look of scorn."

"Okay, let the time move on a few minutes. What's happening?"

"He walks into the other room. I'm sitting there with a book in my hand. I guess I was doing my homework, but I don't feel like doing it now. I feel terrible, angry, hurt, disgusted, I don't know how I feel. Mom comes in and tells me that tomorrow after school I need to get a hair cut. I don't want a hair cut. All the other boys in school have longer hair than me, but she says I have to get a hair cut."

"Let your adult self, with all his wisdom and understanding go back and help your younger self understand."

"That was interesting." Aaron started coming out of trance. "I called him 'father,' but I don't remember ever calling him anything. The only time I can remember him talking, hearing the sound of his voice, was at church. I can't remember him ever talking to me. All I can remember is that disdainful look he would give me, his look of scorn."

"Okay, is there anything else you feel a need to do with your mom or father at this time?" Aaron shook his head no. "Okay, let yourself go back even further in time, being curious and wondering, carrying that mangy feeling with you."

Aaron's trance again deepened and he lifted his finger. "I'm about four years old. I'm sitting in church with mom, sitting where we always sit, in the second row, over to the right. I guess I was squirming around. Mom squeezes my arm. I look up at him in the pulpit and he is giving me his look of scorn. That's the only way he looks at me. He is looking at me like I have the mange."

"Again, let your adult self go back and be with your young self, show your young self that you understand and care, show your young self the love he needs."

Aaron smiled. "Back then he never smiled at me; he always seemed to look at me with a look of scorn. I don't remember his sermons. I don't think I ever listened, but I know he always preached about hell, fire, and brimstone. It was a small church and I think it got smaller as I grew older. Then he retired from the church and opened a Christian book store. He seemed happier there. He always liked books. Though I don't think he wanted me to go to college, even a Christian college, mom wanted me to go. He never said anything to me, let mom do all the talking. I don't remember much about the book store. I guess he started it when I was about 17 years old and I soon went away to college. I'm close to my sister and sometimes mom comes to visit, but my father seems to be a bitter old man. I rarely see him."

THE SHE-BEAST'S AWARENESS

It is not long before Grendel's mother knows someone is exploring her world. In the dissociative process of hypnosis, the client is often surprised by what was remembered or experienced. The experience is as if the memory has a life of its own—as if the client is pulled toward it. This unexpected sense of awareness carries with it a feeling or realization that the experience is very important. The words or affect used as the bridge in this experience are important to understand its significance.

Peggy found the amber lit room, or the room finally found her. Her tormentor was about to carry her away into the realm of the unexpected.

Aaron was carried away by his tormentor when he made the surprising connection between his mangy feeling and his father's scornful look.

Sally was on her way to the bottom of her problem. We had begun time regression using her feelings of anger, disgust, and embarrassment as a bridge. She went back in time to when she was about 14 or 15 years old. Her mother was working second shift, from three to eleven. Sally was at home alone with her step-father. At about 11 P.M. she was in her bedroom studying. She knew her mother would be home in about a half hour, and then she could go to bed. Her parents had divorced when Sally was eight years old. Her father had moved across the country and Sally rarely saw him. She had previously mentioned that her step-father had been a good provider and that she had gotten along with him okay. She called him Bob.

"I am studying on my bed in my bedroom. I am feeling very tired and wish I could go to bed. Bob looks into my room and asks if I shouldn't be getting my shower and getting ready for bed. I tell him I have just a few more pages to read and he leaves. I feel all those feelings, disgust, anger, and embarrassment. I hate it when he looks in on me like that. I'll be glad when mom gets home."

"Let your wise and understanding adult self help your younger self understand."

"Bob makes me feel very uncomfortable. My feelings have something to do with him. Mom loves and needs him. After her divorce from my dad, life was so difficult. She was always worried, and we never seemed to have enough money. She was so unhappy until she met Bob. Now she, we, seem to have what we need, but I don't like Bob. I can't tell her that." Sally knew her tormentor was close at hand and ready for a confrontation.

When Raymond returned for his next session of therapy, we picked up where we had left off. I suggested he go back through time, carrying his neck and shoulder pain with him. His first stop was, "I'm running into the house and the telephone is ringing. I am scared. I know what the phone call is about. One of our neighbors is phoning to tell mom I knocked over their trash cans. We were playing kick the can. I was being chased and I ran around the trash cans and grabbed one of them and knocked it over to get away. I know mom is going to tell me how mad dad is going to be. I yell at her before she gets off the phone, 'I'll pick it all up' and run back out the door."

By this time Raymond had gotten the picture. He knew his problem had something to do with his dad getting mad at him. He was curious. Again, I suggested he go back in time. This time Raymond reported "I just got home from school. I had a math test I flunked. I just didn't understand the assignment. Mom said dad would be very disappointed. When dad got home I ran to him to tell him about the test. He wanted to see it. He was patient and gentle in explaining to me what I didn't understand."

Raymond did not need his dad to be patient and gentle, his dad was patient and gentle. This verified my suspicion that Raymond's mother used the threat that his father would be angry as an attempt to control Raymond, when in fact this threat was empty.

GRABBED BY THE SHE-BEAST

The water hag lunges at Beowulf, grabs him and carries him away. His chainmail protects him from her claws, but while in her clutches, he cannot reach his weapon. Other beasts of this waste-water lake tear at him as she carries him to her den. The defense of his chainmail is effective against them too.

In this world of the unknown, we realize we have found the source of our torment. It grabs us and carries us off, but now we know we have the strength to survive. Our long used defenses were not effective against Grendel, our recently developed problems, but these defenses were built over our lifetime to defend us against the source of our torment.

Raymond began to realize that his mother's threats of his dad's anger were not true. He was soon able to say, "Though dad expected the most of me, he was always patient and gentle. I don't remember him ever getting angry. Mom's threats were wrong. She taught me to fear dad unnecessarily. I felt like I had to do everything to please dad to avoid his anger. That was an unfair trip she put on me."

As we continued with Sally's journey, she began to recall, "If I did take a shower when I was home alone with Bob, he would come into the bathroom, or insist for some stupid reason that I leave the door open. He would sit there on the toilet and watch me, try to talk to me. I would hurry as fast as I could to get to my bedroom. I hated it, the way he looked at me, like a disgusting rat. He has a large, long nose that reminded me of a rat. As long as I was studying, I wouldn't have to get ready for bed. I was so tired so much of the time, studying so late, but I did get good grades. That was the good part of the whole thing—knowing how to study got me through graduate school." Sally was grabbed by the water hag. Her feelings began to fall in place as she recalled and admitted what had happened with Bob.

When we left Craig he was examining the red hanging curtains. He could see a shadowy figure or figures behind them but was unable to identify them. While examining them he began to feel sick to his stomach with anxiety. He was on the trail.

During the next session he journeyed back through time using the sick feelings in his stomach as the bridge. "I am walking in the woods on my grandfather's farm. He is holding my hand and we are walking to the old swimming hole. The swimming hole is just over hill. I've been there many times to watch my cousins swim and play in the water . . . ."

After a short delay I asked, "What's happening now?"

"We get to the hole and my grandfather thinks I should go in. I didn't want to go in. It was too cold and I couldn't swim." Craig demonstrated his resistance by switching to the past tense. He kept an emotional distance from what was going to happen. "He picked me up by the arms and held me over the water. I screamed 'Don't, don't!'"

"He put me down but was angry. 'What do you mean, don't? All boys who visit me have to go swimming! That's what this swimming hole is for! No boy is afraid to go in that hole!' He picked me up again and this time threw me in, yelling, 'The only way to learn to swim is to sink or swim!' I thought I was going to die. I couldn't get my breath and I was coughing. I realized I was standing up in the water. I couldn't move my feet, they were stuck in the mud. I was scared, couldn't catch my breath. I was afraid to get out because he would throw me in again. I was afraid of the water and began to cry.

"He yelled at me, 'cut out that infernal crying! You're being a baby!' I remember crying and being scared. I don't know what happened after that." With the strength of this memory, Grendel's mother had grabbed Craig and was carrying him away.

In preparation for the next step in therapy to help Craig deal with this memory, I suggested, "Let your adult self, with all his wisdom and understanding, go back and give your younger self the understanding and emotional support you need."

As the hypnotic journey continued for Megan, terror and panic grew. She could hear her parents fighting: "I can't stand it; Mom's screaming! Dad too, but he can hardly get his words out. He's not making sense!"

Megan is in a state of panic. I suggested, "Let your adult self go back and comfort your younger self, give her emotional support." Megan is hyperventilating and shaking. I asked, "What is happening?"

"The fight is over and I hear dad coming up the stairs. I'm scared. I can't stand this."

"Let your adult self be with you and comfort you."

"Yeah, she's there, but she's scared too. She's standing over in the corner, scared."

"Okay, let your breathing slow down. Let your breathing become deeper. . . . Take some time to breathe. Inhale calmness. As you exhale, let the calmness flow deeper inside you. Your adult self is ready to face what's happening."

THE SHE-BEAST'S DEN

Upon reaching the beast's den, Beowulf finds he can breathe. Her den is free of water and a fire burns brightly. She carries us home to the source of our torment. Though we have been dissociated from these environs, they hold an unconscious familiarity. This place is not going to destroy or suffocate us. We have been here before and survived. In this world, Beowulf can see, for the first time, the ugliness of the water hag.

When we killed our tormentor Grendel in our own environment, we had no idea from where he came. We had no assurance that the source of our problem was destroyed. By going now to the den of this demon, and killing it at its source, we will know we have prevailed. The demon will not return.

Craig again went back in time, carrying with him the sick feeling in his stomach. This time he was with his cousins and grandfather, walking in the woods toward a rock bluff. Craig was afraid to climb on the rocks and afraid his grandfather was going to get mad at him. Afraid of being afraid, and angry at himself for being afraid, he felt helpless. Craig was now seeing the sea hag clearly in her den.

"Sit there on that rock and look at your grandfather. You feel very afraid of him. Do you have any other feelings?"

"No."

"Think about feeling angry. Does anger seem to fit?"

"No. I can't be angry at him. He's my grandfather."

"Besides being afraid of being afraid, you are afraid of being angry. Think about the deeper feelings of being angry, anger you cannot and will not show. If you saw someone throw a young child in the water, you would feel angry at them though you might not express that anger. You have a right to feel angry at your grandfather. Feeling angry at your grandfather does not mean you would want to hurt him, but you have a right to feel angry."

Craig had faced his tormentor in its den and the struggle had begun.

Megan's father was on his way up the stairs. I continued, "What is happening?"

"Dad is coming into the room. I can hear him breathing hard. He's getting in bed with me. I can't stand this. . . ." She has put her hand over her face and is now sobbing.

Megan's adult self and younger self were both facing the terror of her father getting into bed with her. They had returned to the den of Grendel's mother. Megan's anticipation of this event made it obvious that this had happened before. Megan knew her father was going to get into her bed, but this time she was ready to face it. Her new sense of strength had equipped her to overcome her dissociation of these incidents.

Raymond knows that his dad is patient. I recalled a dream Raymond had brought to therapy weeks before, a dream we considered but left hanging patiently because it did not seem to fit into the picture at the time: "You are walking down a city street when some stranger shouts to you to wait. He scares you and you start walking faster. He is coming after you so you start to run. He starts to run too. You come to the police station and run in. Yet he comes in after you. He hands you your wallet that you had dropped a couple of blocks away. Now that dream makes sense. "You do not need to be afraid of your father."

Raymond had received a clue that he could now understand. He was very familiar with the fear learned in his childhood, but now he was able to understand it clearly. He was in the den of the she-beast.

THE BEGINNING OF THE END

Beowulf swings his sword. It connects with the she-beast's neck, but it does not bite. This precious sword fails in battle for the first time.

The first step in our final battle to overcome our torment is to see it face to face, to relive the original trauma, to respect its strength and to experience our powerlessness against it. Our old weapons bring us to this place but now they fail. Hypnotically recalling and reliving this trauma provides us with this opportunity to face it directly.

In his struggle, Raymond's understanding only causes him to be more resentful of his mother. He sees his tormentor face to face.

Megan was hiding her head under the pillow and pulling tight at her covers when her father got into bed with her. "He is so hot and wet. He stinks of beer. I feel sick to my stomach. He wraps his arm around me and is pressing against my back. I can't stand this. I want to, I'm trying to ignore him. He is breathing so hard, he stinks. I can feel his breath in my ear...."

"What's happening?"

"I feel far away. I hate him there. He's so hot and stinks. I feel far away. He's just laying there, holding me. I think he is crying. At least he's jerking when he breathes. He can't catch his breath."

"Is your adult self still there in the corner?"

"I don't know? I can't see anything. I feel far away."

"Okay, become your adult self. Let your adult self see what's happening. Let your adult self know what's happening."

"Dad is crying. He hurts badly and is just hanging onto me. He scares me."

"Let your adult self see and understand. How is he holding you?"

"He has his arms round my stomach. He's holding me tight. He's so hot, pressing against me."

Though it may have made little difference, I wondered if this embrace was sexual. "Let your adult self help you find the words to describe what he is doing."

"He is just holding me. He's scared and hurt. I feel suffocated. He stinks."

"What is he wearing?"

"Oh, he's wearing his plaid shirt and jeans, like he wears most the time."

At this point I assumed this incident was not sexual; yet Megan's father was using his daughter for emotional support, emotional incest.

Peggy finally arrived at the amber lit bedroom. She felt strange and different. She talks slowly, "I'm a teenager, 15 or 16 years old. My hair is blond. This is strange. This room is real old. The mattress is lumpy, I think it is filled with straw. It's high off the floor. I'm wearing a white or off white nightgown or slip. The material is sort of rough, . . . lying on the bed." Peggy was panting, hyperventilating. "I'm scared. I'm screaming." She put her fist to her mouth and bit on her knuckles. "Nobody can hear me. My husband is gone, somewhere out in the fields. He's too far away. I'm in pain. I'm pregnant, in labor. I can't breathe. The bed feels all wet, I think its blood. I can't see. I'm scared. I feel dizzy, like I'm going to pass out. . . ."

"Peggy! Go back and be with your other self. You can be there for her. You are in labor. What's your name?"

"Mary Elizabeth."

"Mary Elizabeth, Peggy is there for you, Peggy is there to help you. She knows what is going on, she knows you, she is you . . . What is going on?"

Peggy answered. "She is laying there quiet. She passed out. She is very white. I think she is about to die. She's not suffering now. She seems so peaceful."

Peggy's hypnotic journey took her to what has been called a past life. The importance of this experience is that she found a life's trauma that has been affecting her current life situation. This trauma, found in the context of a past life experience, was unexpected, a surprise, but it was effective, as we will see, providing her relief from her current problems. Who am I to say that this experience was not a real experience from a past life? It may have been. It may also have been a metaphoric reliving of some current traumatic life experience, a life experience too painful for her to face more directly. Peggy's shrug of the shoulders, no big deal attitude, was used on several occasions in therapy to brush aside her father's abandonment of the family when she was only one year old. This issue had never been faced, or maybe it was being faced metaphorically in this past life experience. In either case, this experience offered Peggy a means to deal with the trauma and a way to heal on her journey to living a more effective life.

Aaron had found the mangy mutt side of himself, the look of scorn his father would give him. Now was the time to face that look in all its intensity. During the last session Aaron showed some ability to dissociate from the emotional pain of that look by examining it with pure curiosity as if it were outside of himself. "Go back and be with your younger self sitting in church with your mother. You look up to see your father giving you a look of scorn. You saw his scornful look many other times too. See him looking at you. Feel that look entering you. Let that feeling sink deep within you. Feel the disgust you feel with his look of scorn, feel the disgust within you. Hold on to it. Think of other times when he looked at you that way."

Aaron described another incident. "My sister is four years older than me. She wanted a new dress for her junior high school graduation and showed a picture of one from an ad in the paper to mom. My father showed his look of scorn. I think probably the dress only had straps over the shoulders or something like that. But father said, 'What do you think Aaron would think if he saw you dressed like that?' He gave me a scornful look, too. I remember feeling confused, not knowing what I would think."

"Let your wise and understanding adult self go back and help your younger self understand."

"He was thinking it looked too sexy, but I wasn't even thinking about sex yet. I didn't know what he was talking about."

"Let your wise and understanding adult self go back and help your other younger selves understand."

"When I was in church I really don't remember why mom squeezed my arm. I just assumed it was because I was squirming because that is what kids do. When I wanted to let my hair grow long like other kids in school, I didn't understand why I needed to get it cut. I think I might have even told Mom 'Jesus had long hair,' I know I thought that years later when I was in college. It was a Christian college and all the guys wore dress shirts and ties and had short hair. I thought it was ridiculous and remembered mentioning that Jesus had long hair to some of my friends."

THE WARRIOR AND BEAST GRAPPLE

Beowulf doesn't loose heart but grabs the beast with his hand and throws her to the ground. She immediately rises and grabs him, flinging him to the ground.

She unsheathes her dagger and attempts to stab him, but her dagger cannot penetrate his chainmail.

Once the original trauma is uncovered hypnotically, the second step toward victory over this she-beast is to grapple with her, to face her with bare hands, to grapple with the original trauma with an immediate sense of reality, identifying totally with the feelings of the experience. One useful technique is to suggest that the adult self, with all its wisdom and understanding, go back and be with the younger self. This adult self understands better than anyone else what this younger self felt and helps this younger self find the right words to describe how she or he felt in the traumatic situation. A child generally has not learned the words to describe feelings and the parent often does not have the understanding or patience to teach the child these words at the time of the trauma. Using the words of feelings can give a person a greater sense of control over the appropriate feelings.

Peggy identified her terror, her pain and panic. She uncovered the amber lit room in a "past life," in a situation where she needed someone to help her and no one came.

Aaron was able to find the right words to describe his feelings. He dissociated somewhat from his feelings of having mange but recalled more clearly feeling confused, thinking that his father was "ridiculous." He was able to identify his feelings of being "hurt and humiliated" by his father's disdainful look, and maybe "embarrassed," but he thought his father should have felt more embarrassed to be giving him that look from the pulpit. Aaron had the strength, even as an adolescent, to resent his father, but he admitted that he had felt "unloved" by his father. "Even now I feel my father loves nobody. I'm not even sure he loves God. He never loved me. I think my mother did her best to love me, but I don't think he approved of her loving me."

"How about God? Imagine God looking down on you. What's God's expression?"

"Scornful. Why would anybody believe in such a God?"

Sally felt disgusted, angry, embarrassed, and afraid of Bob. Over a period of three therapy sessions, more and more of what happened from when she was 14 to 16 years old came back. She reported she knew what had happened, but the memory was vague; she didn't want to admit it; it seemed almost unreal. During one session, with hypnotic regression, Sally recalled "One night after I took a shower, I hurried and got into bed." Her use of past tense put this experience one step removed from reliving it, making it easier for her to recall. "It was only about nine o'clock but I was especially tired and had a test the next day. I needed my sleep more than I needed to study. Bob came into my bedroom and got into my bed. He had no clothes on. He, he put his arms around me and slipped his hand under my nightgown. . . ." Sally was sobbing and could not go on.

"Your adult self knows how you feel better than anyone else, she knows you survived this awful time. Let her go back and be with your younger self. She can tell your younger self you did nothing wrong. You know Bob has big problems.

You have every right to hate him, to be afraid of him. . . ." I waited quietly a few minutes and Sally began to calm down.

When she opened her eyes I told her, "You did a good job. It's very scary to admit this to yourself. You don't know now what you are going to do with it. You see this kind of thing so much in your work, but when it is you, it is terrifying. You may need to come back to what happened over and over, but you will do it only as you are emotionally ready to do it. You were emotionally ready to face it today. You are much stronger than you were before. You have come a long way. You don't know what you need to do about these memories. Should you tell your mother? There is no reason to make this decision right away. What's more important first is for you to deal with your own feelings, and find the strength within you to help you make the decision. You have had much experience working with other people in situations not much different from yours. You have all the time you need. Now is the time to let yourself feel the disgust, anger, embarrassment and fear of Bob. There is no need to see him or face him right now. You do talk to your mother and you may have a hard time talking to her this week." We then discussed what she might say to her mother, for example: "If I seem different or seem like something is bothering me, I am working on something in therapy. When the time is right I will tell you about it. Right now I need to do some work on it for myself. Thank you for being patient with me."

Sally explained that when she was 16 and molested by Jake, her mother was called at work and came and got her from school. When Bob heard the story he was horrified about what Jake had done and threatened to kill him, but Bob never sexually abused her again. For the last 17 years their relationship had been cordial, but not close.

Raymond had realized that his father was indeed patient and gentle. His fear of his father had been created only from the words of his mother.

I suggested, "With this new-found wisdom of your adult self, go back and help your younger self understand, help your younger self find the appropriate feeling for this new understanding."

"I feel ripped off by Mom. I had no reason to fear Dad and I don't fear him when I'm with him, only when I do something wrong and think about him. I resent this trip Mom put on me all these years; she had no right to deceive me like this. I've spent a lot of my life worrying about what Dad would think. What a waste of energy! It wasn't fair. I spent so much energy trying to please Dad so he wouldn't be mad. What Mom said was not real. Knowing this takes so much responsibility off my shoulders."

Raymond and I both laughed—he knew what I was thinking.

In pursuing the feelings of Megan, the most dominant feeling was one of suffocation. As she went on, she identified feeling trapped. Her father had been looking for emotional support and love, using her as a surrogate wife, and she also felt confused. On the one hand she had sought to be close to him. After all, he was her father. Yet he didn't know how to be close. By identifying the appropriate words to describe what she felt, she found greater control over her feelings.

FINDING THE NEEDED WEAPON

Beowulf sees, stashed in the cave, a prized sword forged by the giants. This sword, famous for winning many battles, is too heavy to be lifted by most men. Beowulf seizes it and swings, severing the head of the water hag. As her head falls, the cave fills with light. Beowulf sees the corpse of Grendel. To settle accounts he severs the head of this lifeless body.

Beowulf finds the needed instrument to win his battle. In our battle against our tormentor, what is our need? If the source of our battle is with a parent who is insensitive to our needs or who does not trust us or shows us no respect, we can tell this parent what we need: "Mom, I need you to be more understanding of my feelings. Dad, I need you to be patient and respect me." It is easy to say how we don't want to be: "I'm never going to beat my children," or "I'm not going to keep them from their friends." But it is much more difficult to define how we want to be.

"Let the wise and understanding adult self go back and be with your younger self and help your younger self find the right words to state what you needed from you mother or father." Just as Beowulf finds his needed weapon, we need to arm our inner child with the necessary weapon of naming what the child needs from the parent. Children generally lack both the language ability or the perspective to state what they need. Our adult self can provide this language and perspective for our inner child. In speaking these words hypnotically we are speaking to the inner mother or inner father, that conception we hold within regarding what a mother or a father means to us. By speaking to the inner mother or inner father, we heal or integrate that aspect of ourselves; our motherly and fatherly roles become healthy.

With this hypnotic experience of understanding what we need, we are on the way to victory; the cave lights up our awareness of the source of our torment. In this light we see the connection between this experience and our original tormentor, Grendel. We now make sure Grendel is dead.

Sally needed to talk to her father archetype, telling him what she needed. I gave her a homework assignment of listing these needs beginning with some suggestions—"Bob (and/or dad, and/or Bart), I need to be able to trust you to be sensitive to my needs, to my feelings. I need you to respect my needs. I need you to be gentle with me and protect me from things that frighten, disgust, or hurt me." These suggestions, however, were only a beginning and would need to be defined and clarified. Sally's father archetype was mixed up with Bob, her abandoning father, Bart, and her expectations of a father and of men in general. She needed to address these comments inward to help heal her expectations of an inner father figure, and, in doing so, address it by the name that seemed to her to fit the best. Still, the light had come on, and she was able to connect this hypnotic experience to her Grendel and make certain it was dead.

Craig had begun to define the feelings that lay behind his obsessive worry. He had started by defining his need to please and his fear of upsetting others. He had now begun to grapple with the deeper feelings, not only his fear of disappointing his grandfather, but also his anger toward and resentment of his grandfather for not allowing him to be afraid.

To take Craig beyond these feelings of fear and anger, it was important to lead him to define what he needed from his grandfather and from others, especially men, in his life. I asked Craig to have his wise and understanding adult self go back and help his younger self understand what he needed from his grandfather. I offered the suggestions, "Grandpa, I need you to allow me my feelings, to let me feel afraid, and to offer me emotional support when I am afraid."

Craig was able to go further with specific examples. "Grandpa, when I am afraid of the water, I need you to be gentle, gentle in carrying me into the water. I need you to show me how much fun it is to play in the water. When I climb rocks I need you to be gentle in showing me how to do it." Craig had later learned to swim and had even become a summer swimming instructor when he was in college. He knew very well how important it was for children to enjoy the water while learning, and that to teach a child to enjoy water, the instructor needs to be gentle.

I asked Craig to take this experience further by thinking of and writing down other incidents of others being insensitive to his feelings. Then, he could write down his needs in these situations, writing them in as many different ways as he could. By clarifying his needs, Craig had seen the light and could now say with certainty that his Grendel was dead.

Megan's needs included, "I need Dad to respect me and to allow me to be carefree. I need Dad to love Mom and allow me to feel secure in their love. I need Dad to stay sober. I also need to be able to trust Dad with my feelings, to talk to him about what is important to me and know he will be understanding and patient."

What were Peggy's needs? "I need someone to be there with me. I need support in my pain and struggle. I need the one I love to be there, to demonstrate love by being there in my time of greatest need."

Aaron said, "I need my father to love me. I need a father who can appreciate me and love me."

"Can you say that again as if you were talking to your father, the father within you?"

"Father, I need you to show me you love me. I need you to appreciate me and try to understand how I think and feel."

"The word 'father' sounds so cold. Think about how you felt when you watched Nan. You felt warm. If you had a son think about what you would want him to call you."

"Yeah, I would hope he would call me Dad or Daddy."

"Try again to talk to the dad or daddy within you."

"Dad, I need you to show me you love me and appreciate me. I need to have you understand my feelings about things, my feelings when other kids in school have long hair and mine is short. Dad, I need you to let me be me."

Raymond needed "Mom to be honest and teach me that Dad is gentle and patient. I need to trust Dad to be gentle and patient as a father should."

Victory was at hand.

HROTHGAR RETURNS HOME

From the shore Hrothgar and his men see the blood boiling in the lake. After nine hours, they feel certain Beowulf must be dead. They give up their wait to return to Heorot, leaving Beowulf's men on the shore alone.

Though we have experienced the death of Grendel and his mother, we still have not experienced a sense of real change within us. We sometimes become impatient or discouraged and give up waiting to experience the real change. However, part of us continues to have patience and faith. The process of change takes some time and requires repeatedly facing our tormentor in as many different experiences and situations as possible, repeatedly identifying our feelings about each situation, and repeatedly identifying our needs in each situation. This can be done in therapy and also through the homework assignment of journaling. At times this process may become discouraging. Sometimes the emotional pain is such that a client needs to take some time out from the healing process. Sometimes it takes an extra amount of emotional support from significant others in one's life, or from others with similar experiences as can occur in group therapy or support groups.

Craig knew he needed others to be gentle with him and allow him his feelings, but when they didn't, he felt even more overwhelmed by his obsessive worry. Hardly a day would go by at work when someone wouldn't come to him with a complaint; listening to complaints was part of his job. Yet because of the nature of his job, he could not tell these people he was overwhelmed by their complaints. His duty was to find a solution and get them what they wanted. Now, rather than think how he could screw up the work or what he might do to displease others, with each demand or complaint he would think, "I need someone to hold me, someone to understand how stressed I am by all these complaints or demands." He became even more supersensitive to how others were insensitive to him. Almost everyone was ignoring his feelings and expecting him to meet their needs. He felt discouraged by what he thought was his victory. He was ready to leave the lake and return to the safety of his home.

Raymond was talking of what he needed from his mother: "I need mom to be honest with me and to teach me that dad is patient and gentle. Mom, I need you to be loving and strong and not pass the buck to dad." Raymond wondered if this situation had something to do with his inability to delegate at work and not share feelings at home.

I suggested that Raymond had learned to not trust "passing the buck" because part of him knew his mother did it dishonestly.

When Megan first identified her needs, she became more angry at her father and wanted to hurt him. She needed his respect but she didn't respect him. He had caused her so much pain; he was so weak. Her King within was discouraged and left to return home to safety.

BEOWULF GATHERS THE EVIDENCE

The fiery blood of the she-beast dissolves the sword into a puddle of melted iron. Though Beowulf can see great treasures in the cave, he takes nothing from this den except the jeweled handle of the sword and Grendel's head. Death of these monsters purifies the lake, and light shines in.

For final reassurance of our victory we need to gather up its evidence. We do not gather the other treasures, nor focus on other victories, because at that moment they would be a distraction from this victory. We focus on and gather evidence for this victory alone. We need to see that the archetypes within us, our mother archetype and our father archetype, are whole, integrated into healthiness. We can see this best in our relationships with others. Has our ability to mother and father our own children, to father and mother our spouse or parents, to father and mother our employees grown, and become healthy and whole? We begin collecting evidence by noticing the changes in the way we relate to others.

Raymond had been successful this last year while practicing "passing the buck" in an honest manner. These pieces were coming together, becoming more the real Raymond.

Megan spent considerable time in therapy expressing anger at her father. I frequently came back to her needs—her need for her father to respect her and to support her in being carefree. We came back to her need for her father to be patient and listen to what was important to Megan, for her father to love her mother so Megan could be free of the responsibility to fill her father's need for love, and for her to feel secure in her parent's love for each other. I asked her to find within herself the ability to support others' need to be carefree and the ability to feel security in her own love of her husband. With a father who felt unloved by her mother, how could she reassure her husband of her love?

Megan and her husband were hoping to have children, but they had put off this decision until Megan's depression was resolved. I suggested that Megan imagine having a child, an infant. "What does it mean to respect an infant?"

"If he or she cries, listen and try to understand why he or she is crying."

"That takes a lot of patience."

"I know. I babysat some in high school. I would become so frustrated."

"Go back to when you babysat and the baby is crying. You feel so frustrated, you could scream. Is it a boy or a girl?"

"A girl."

"You feel so frustrated you could scream at her. Maybe you keep your cool, maybe you don't, but if you don't, the baby feels your tension. Your tension scares the baby causing her to cry more. Take a few moments to regain your sense of calm. Look at her, listen to her with a calm sense of curiosity and strength. She is whimpering but not crying out of control. Let your confident sense of curiosity grow. Notice your feeling of frustration disappears. The baby becomes quiet. You are able to respect her need to cry.

"Now, do the same thing with your husband. He is not listening to you or understanding you. You feel so frustrated. But, now, take a few minutes to feel a quiet sense of curiosity grow within you. Feel yourself gaining a sense of strength and personal power with this quiet curiosity. With your sense of curiosity you are respecting your husband's feelings. He then calms down and is able to respect your feelings. When you are frustrated, his frustration builds. Now, with mutual respect and curiosity, you both can listen to each other. Take time to practice this next week. It will be very good preparation for having a baby."

Megan had the opportunity to learn to be for herself what she needed from her father. When she becomes this new, healed person, she will have the emotional strength to let go of her anger at her father. Megan will be collecting the evidence to prove to herself her victory.

Aaron had discovered his need to feel loved by his father: "I need to have him look at me with a look of love, a gentle look of love." Aaron was still struggling with the need to feel loved. He needed to collect evidence that he was loved and able to love. "Go back and let yourself be with your niece. You are at one of the family get-togethers with your sister and her family. Look at Nan, your niece, with a sense of loving support. Feel your love flow from you and watch her respond, watch her respond to you in a loving way. Do the same thing with your wife. Look at her with a look of love and watch her look back at you with love. By just being loving, people will love you, you will feel lovable. Take credit for being loving and lovable. Now imagine your father looking at you with that scornful look. This may be difficult at first, but see if you can melt that look of scorn by looking at him with love. You have every right to be angry at him, and you may not be ready to melt his look of scorn with your look of love, but just keep the idea in mind. Someday you will be ready."

Aaron was collecting evidence of his ability to love and be loved.

Peggy, whether from an actual experience from a past life, or from a metaphoric expression of some trauma in her current life too painful to face directly, needed loving support from a significant other. She felt this support from her boyfriend with whom she now spent many nights, but this relationship was still new with no commitment for the future. She believed she had loving support from her mother, but her experience in therapy suggested she needed to feel loving support within herself. To nurture the feeling within herself, she needed to offer this loving support to others. Peggy's job as a paralegal placed her in daily situations where others needed loving support. Though her boyfriend seemed to be strong and psychologically healthy, there were times when he also needed loving support. I asked Peggy to let her therapy experience change her to be to others what she had needed from her husband in her hypnotic "past life" experience.

Peggy returned to therapy the next week with a perfect example and experience. She reported working on a child custody case in which the father had kidnaped the children. Her client had not seen the children for over a month. "The mother was in tears, actually beating her chest, hurting for not seeing her children. I gave her a hug and just held her. There was nothing I could or needed to say. We were already doing everything we could to get the kids back."

Peggy was able to provide the loving support she needed for herself.

To heal the needy part of ourselves we need to apply our healing energy to others. When we do so, we collect personal evidence of change.

166 / GRENDEL AND HIS MOTHER

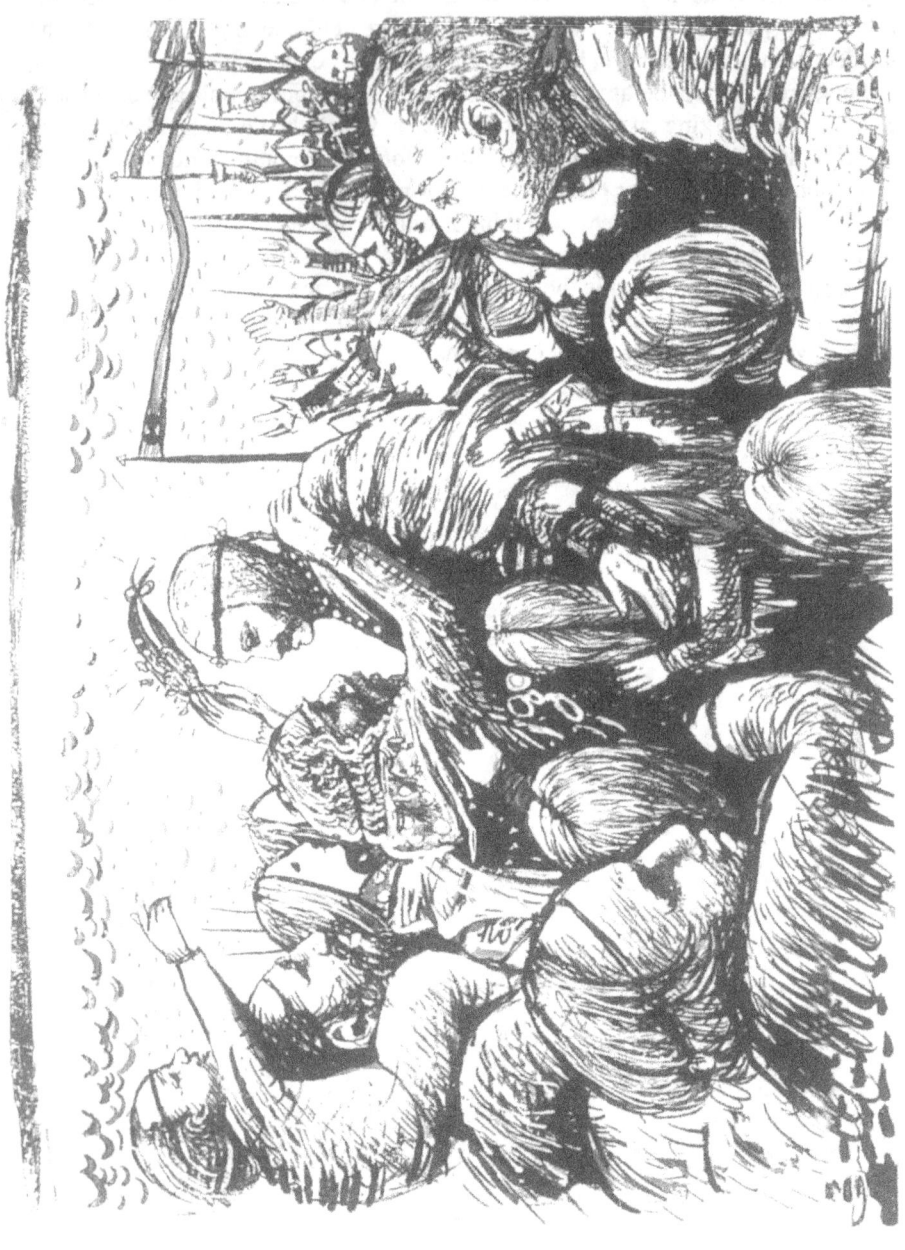

CHAPTER X

The Final Celebration

Beowulf swims ashore to be greeted with relief and excitement by the other warriors in his party. From the shore of the lake he returns to Heorot to seek an audience first with the Queen and then with the King. A parallel to this event is the performer of a great athletic feat who is first greeted by his teammates and then embraced by his mother before receiving a hug and slap on the back from his father.

When we examine our internal archetypes, we first are greeted by our internal warriors or "teammates," for they know better than anyone else the significance of our feat. We clench and shake our fists to ourselves in strength and chant "I did it!" or "I made it!" The warrior part of us cheers. We then consider the vulnerable but nurturing femaleness within ourselves. We are amazed at ourselves for going beyond our usual vulnerability and feel even more proud and appreciative of how we protected this vulnerable part of us. Finally, we face the king within, the wise and understanding part of ourselves, to put the whole incident in perspective, to challenge us to not become overconfident but to remain humble and prudent in our victory.

BEOWULF SWIMS ASHORE

Thanking God, Beowulf's 13 remaining gallant men are delighted to see Beowulf swim ashore. Our warrior self, that part of us who faced our tormentor and overcame it, is delighted in the victory and needs to celebrate.

Aaron felt victorious. When he looked at his wife he could feel the warmth of his love; he could smile. When he looked at his niece, Nan, he would feel warmth and could smile when she smiled at him. The smiles became infectious and the warmth grew. He spent a lot of time laughing and feeling light-hearted.

Peggy found and faced the amber lit room in a "past life" experience. She realized her need for someone to love her and be there for her. Rationally, she believed she had loving support from her mother and boyfriend, yet she had felt alone and frightened much of the time. But when she showed others loving support, she felt more fully loved by others. Peggy had experienced a great victory and was swimming ashore. As she explained, "I feel like a new person. I am looking at the world differently, feeling love where before I felt insecure."

Raymond felt cheated by his mother's threat that his father would be angry or disappointed because of his wrongdoings or mistakes. Raymond was gentle and patient with his own children, and now he wondered briefly if his wife ever used the threat of his punishment with their children. But he couldn't imagine she would use this threat, and he agreed it wasn't her style.

Raymond now understood the source of his irritability. As he learned in childhood to seek to please his father, he became a perfectionist. When life was not perfect, he would become irritable. When especially stressed, as when he moved and was promoted, his irritability would become obvious to others. Now he had gone through the four steps of healing. First, he identified the "trauma": his mother's threats of punishment from his father. Second, he identified the resulting feelings: fear, followed by feeling "ripped off" or cheated by his mother, and frustrated for never having appreciated the gentle and patient nature of his father. Third, he stated his needs of his mother and father in positive terms: "Mom, I need you to be honest and teach me that dad is gentle and patient. I need to trust dad to be patient and gentle." Fourth, he recognized these needed behaviors in himself. He had always tried to be patient and gentle with his children, but he would become irritable though he tried not to show it. He now felt a new level of patience and gentleness. Moreover, he became much more "patient and gentle" with his employees. Raymond was experiencing the benefits of his victory. He was coming ashore.

As Raymond enjoyed this success, we talked about how he might talk to his parents. As he felt more confident in himself, his resentment of his mother diminished. He realized, at least intellectually, that she did what she felt she needed to do at the time and really was a good mother. We decided he could question her, with a sense of curiosity, about why she used the threat of punishment from his father as a means of control. With Raymond's new-found ability to be gentle and patient, he was able to talk to his mother about this subject without causing her to become defensive or deny her childrearing tactic.

Raymond's mother talked about how strict her father had been and how she had feared him. Still, she thought that in meting out spankings, he was more fair than her mother, who would just yell and scream. She did not want to be a yeller and screamer like her mother, so she tried to stay calm when she had to discipline the children. She felt frustrated at times because Raymond's father seemed to her too gentle or patient. Even though she thought he let the children get away with too much, she realized that the children were generally good children, so she was satisfied with this arrangement. By turning the punishment over to Raymond's father, she was able to stay calm and not be like her mother.

Raymond understood and appreciated the talk he had with his mother. He had come ashore to celebrate.

Sally now knew why she would go into a rage when Brad would watch her dressing or undressing. At first it seemed to be because of the incident in high school when Jake grabbed her breast, but dealing with that incident was not enough. Then she began to remember her step-father's behavior, the way he would come into the bathroom when she was bathing and the way he would insist she leave the bathroom door open. Eventually she remembered his getting into bed with her and fondling her. With time, she remembered this one incident in greater detail. Her step-father did not penetrate her sexually, but pressed against her from behind and did ejaculate. Sally was disgusted, angry, and embarrassed. The incident was never talked about, and when the incident with Jake happened, her step-father was horrified and never harassed her sexually again.

Sally knew how much her mother had needed her step-father. I had suggested to her there was nothing further she needed to do until she felt stronger, or healed, in dealing with the abuse. As therapy continued, she felt more and more certain that she could not tell her mother what had happened or confront her step-father. She identified her needs for gentleness, protection, and respect, and found that these needs were met by her husband. Sally could relate to Brad with respect and gentleness, and protect him from her rage. Brad's respect for her likewise grew.

Since her step-father had not assaulted or harassed her for all the years since she was 16 years old, and in fact had been a supportive father-figure while she was in college, she continued to see no need to confront him or upset her mother's relationship with him. She did not need for him to say anything. She knew he "felt very bad" about what he had done.

I offered, "I respect your decision. But if for some reason, your feelings change and you feel you need to do something, I'll do what I can to help." Sally came ashore from her victory feeling strong in her decision and in her new understanding, offering her own mother the protection and respect she had needed from her.

THE RETURN TO HEOROT AND QUEEN WEALHTHEOW

Beowulf's men laboriously carry the hilt of the giant's sword and Grendel's head on a spear back to the great hall. Upon arriving, they salute Hrothgar and carry the head of Grendel across the hall filled with celebrating Danes to present before the Queen.

We need to present our victory to the receptive, nurturing, and vulnerable part of ourselves, our inner Queen or femaleness. It is this vulnerable part of ourselves we rose to protect. From this part of ourselves we are most amazed by our strength and victory. This soft and receptive part of ourselves protected us by offering a safe but hidden bed chamber. Now we can assure this protective part of ourselves that we will be safe anywhere.

Sally greatly appreciated Bart for staying at her side during all these months of struggle. She had always been able to see how her volatile feelings had confused and upset him, but now she understood where these feelings had come from. Now that she understood herself and the repressed issues causing her volatility, she could spend time nurturing and caring for her own wounds. Setting aside the anger and humiliation caused by her step-father, she also nurtured her mother by not confronting her or her step-father. At last she was ready to nurture and care for Bart. Having grown in nurturance and sensitivity, Sally had found her healthy inner queen/mother.

Addressing his Queen Wealhtheow, Raymond, too, became more nurturing and sensitive to himself as well as to others around him. He now accepted the gentleness of his father and understood the reason for his mother's threat of punishment from his father. He had learned a lot about his family and himself, and as a result he became a much better parent, husband and employer. The nurturing and sensitive queen within came alive.

When we last met Craig he was feeling quite discouraged. He had discovered that he needed others to understand him, to allow him to express his feelings and to be gentle with him, as he had needed his grandfather to do. Now Craig was discouraged because no one in his life met his needs, especially at work where others expected him to solve their problems.

He needed to collect the evidence of his victory before swimming ashore and meeting the queen. He needed to be for himself what his grandfather wasn't: to be the nurturing and sensitive queen/mother. He needed to give himself permission to be afraid, to cry, and to be angry. Before expecting others to be sensitive and understanding to him, Craig needed to be sensitive and understanding of others as well as himself.

Craig had every right to be angry at his grandfather, father, and mother. He had a right to be angry at his father for being impossible to please and at his mother for saying to his brother, "Why can't you be more like Craig?" His anger had found a way of expression through his fantasies of defiance and rebellion—qualities he envied in his brother but feared in himself.

Now all the pieces came together for Craig's audience with the king, but first he needed to collect the evidence of his victory. He needed to express his feelings of fear and, especially, anger, both within himself, and toward his parents and grandfather. Craig had been experiencing his four-year-old son's current stage of development, a stage of defiance and anger, a stage for developing autonomy. His son's behavior provided a useful teaching experience. I suggested, "Watch your son during one of his tantrums. Appreciate his energy in seeking greater autonomy. Then lovingly give him a hug, without resenting his expression of feelings. Be to your son what your grandfather was not to you." With this exercise, Craig found his ability to be sensitive and understanding of other people's feelings. He found the nurturing queen/mother within.

At the end of the last session with Megan, after the hypnotic role play of holding an infant, I asked her if there were any infants in her life.

"The receptionist in our office has a 9-month-old daughter."

"Can you spend some time with them and hold the baby?"

"I guess so. They are neighbors and we see them occasionally."

"Good. Do what we did today. Hold the baby, listening with curiosity and see what happens. Try this with your husband too." Hopefully Megan would have the nurturing experience of holding and quieting a baby.

THE AUDIENCE WITH THE KING

Beowulf then offers a speech to King Hrothgar—"We bring you the spoils from the lake. By God's grace, I barely escaped death in my underwater battle but found victory by killing the defender of hell. You can now sleep carefree in Heorot."

We next carry the news of our success to the wise and understanding part of ourselves which gives us assurance of our victory. That part of ourselves in return frees us from responsibility to defend him.

Craig completed the full circle of his victory by expressing his feelings of anger and resentment for his parents and grandfather. He resented them for teaching him his obsessive need to please, his need for perfection and his inability to express anger. He understood why he envied his brother's defiance and rebellion. By appreciating his son's emotional expression, he accepted his own expression of anger and resentment. In this way, Craig became free to be himself and to find his own autonomy in emotional expression. When he told the wise and understanding king within of his victory, the king understood and believed.

Peggy's life and therapy experiences of this last year had offered her the relief she sought to be able to wake in the morning rested. Such experiences are most important in facilitating change, but understanding of what caused the change gives the person the tools to help in the future, the King's wisdom.

I summarized for Peggy, "In searching for the trauma in your life that caused you to have nightmares, you found in a past life the amber lit room where you died terrified because your husband wasn't there when you needed him. You felt abandoned by him. The fear of abandonment, whether in your past life or in this life, caused you apprehension in this life. I can't help but think of your father whom you lost when your were one-year-old. But whatever the loss, what you need is loving care from a male figure who will be there for you. To be assured of such love you need to find this constant love in yourself, to show constant love to others. You are beginning to experience this love and, with time, it will be yours."

During the sessions presented in the previous chapter, Megan used imagery to role play babysitting a crying baby. When she learned to respect and understand the baby's cry, this new attitude quickly quieted the baby. Megan then used the same attitude when communicating with her husband, and with practice she became proficient. She discovered she had the sensitivity and nurturing ability of the Queen in many situations. What she did not understand was what this nurturing ability had to do with her father and husband. I began an hypnotic monologue:

"When your father was crying and hurt, when your father got in bed with you, you were a young girl and should not have been expected to be the sensitive and nurturing mother or wife to your father. You were too young and too afraid and confused to nurture him the way he wanted. The wise part of you knew what you had to do. You escaped from the situation in your own head because it was too frightening and painful. The part of you who could care for and nurture a man died in the process. You know how to care for and nurture infants and children, you showed that last week, and you can, if you try hard, nurture and care for your husband, but it is more difficult because those unconscious feelings of fear and pain come back when you are expected to care for and nurture a man, especially an adult man. But what has died is coming back to life. With some understanding and practice, with the understanding that your husband is not your weak and drunken father, you can nurture him."

With this speech, Megan understood, and the wise and understanding king came alive within her.

Aaron also took his victory to the king. He had not had an extramarital affair for nearly two years except for the relapse at the conference and the subsequent cyberaffair. He gave up that affair with little problem and regained his loving and protective status with his wife, sister, and niece. He came at last to thrive on their emotional support and love, an experience of love broader than just a sexual love.

As Aaron's understanding of love grew, he had another insight regarding his father. "My father does not comprehend the meaning of love. He uses fear of hell and damnation to save him from going astray from mom. That is not love. The gospel of love is foreign to him."

Aaron is valuing the warmer, protective love of a healthy relationship with the women in his life. But I still do not completely trust this growth. He still prefers to be in the company of women and has little to do with men. Drawn to seek the attention of women, he may still be vulnerable to extramarital affairs.

THE KING'S ORATION

King Hrothgar examines the hilt of the great sword and warns Beowulf of the importance of being prudent and humble, challenging him to be different than Heremod, an ancient and infamous tyrant king of Denmark. "God grants wisdom and rank to men of noble race. To these men, misfortune is unknown until, in their conceit and arrogance, they take the grace of God for granted and drop their guard for the attack of the devil. Be on guard against such wickedness." Hrothgar uses his own life as an example, "After fifty years of great fortune I did not expect this enemy to cause such suffering."

The king within sets us free from what has tormented us, challenges us to maintain our guard and beseeches us to be prudent and humble. Though we have every right to be proud, we cannot allow ourselves to believe this is our final battle. We need to be continually vigilant for possible future tormentors.

Megan now understood the death of her depression and the rebirth of her ability to care for and nurture a man. Yet this rebirth needed to grow and mature. She needed practice to listen to and respect the feelings of her husband. On the one hand, he was not the infant whom she had learned to listen to and respect. On the other, he was an adult whose nurturance and protection her needy part still craved. She was cautioned that maturity would take work and practice. Though she had the necessary insight, her new expectations of herself still felt strange. With this feeling of strangeness, the King within was offering her words of caution.

Raymond was a very practical man. He had been a perfectionist and always sought to please his father. During our last session, from his practical side he asked, "Will my tension come back? I thought it was gone, but then it came back with the downsizing. Do you think it's gone for good this time?"

My answer to him was, "Your neck and shoulder pain was a sign from your unconscious mind that something was wrong. It was an important sign that you need to value because it gave you the direction and motivation to change. You are on a life long journey of change and personal growth. I hope and expect that you will get other signs from your unconscious mind when you are ready for the next step of growth. It may be neck and shoulder pain. It may be some other sign, but listening for and following these signs are important." Raymond received the message that he needs to be humble and listen to the inner king's orations.

Aaron paraded his victory in front of the Queen and took his story to the King. His newfound feelings of love, warmth, smiles, and laughter were most infectious when around the women in his extended family. He felt he could love them and they loved him. His sensitive, nurturing, and vulnerable side had been wounded but now felt healed. Yet he experienced little feeling with regard to his brother-in-law. They talked about "men's things," about work and home repairs. Occasionally they talked about sports, but with little feeling. He felt neither a need to impress nor a feeling of superiority to his brother-in-law. To Aaron, at family gatherings his brother-in-law was little more than just there. When it came to his father, Aaron would just as soon avoid him. When he was near him, the feelings ranged from negative to nothing.

I felt it was necessary for Aaron to face the meaning of men in his life. It so happened that the next weekend Aaron participated in a gathering of the whole family. Aaron was in one room with his sister, his niece Nan, his mother, and Sandy. Bill, his brother-in-law, was in another room with Aaron's father. As he interacted with the women, Aaron was full of ebullience. Then the two men came in from the other room and caught Aaron laughing and carrying on. When in the past Aaron would have become silent in his father's presence, this time he kept on laughing. He did not feel suffocated by his father's wet blanket. He kept laughing and smiling in front of his father who responded with his customary look of scorn. This interchange struck Aaron as funny, even ridiculous, prompting him to laugh and smile even more.

Soon after, Aaron and his wife were with his sister and Bill. Aaron talked about the family gathering and how he felt his ebullience tormented his father. Aaron explained that he found the situation hilarious and that he enjoyed tormenting his father, getting even with him for all the years of feeling hurt and humiliated.

Bill mentioned that he had noticed Aaron's father's response, too, and added that if anything could "loosen up" his father-in-law it would be Aaron's smiles and laughter.

For once Aaron heard a deeper side of Bill. He felt complimented by Bill's comment. As he laughed with Bill, Aaron felt a positive connection with another man, a feeling of another man's respect for him.

Until this point in his victory over the water hag, Aaron seemed to relate only to women. Now he found that with his new feelings of self-respect, he could at last feel the respect of other men. With this revelation, Aaron took his victory to the King, his wise and insightful self, who also showed him respect.

Aaron acknowledged the change in his life but knew he needed to continue to be ready for further challenges and changes. The feeling of respect from his brother-in-law surprised him, and he realized how much he valued it. Though he evidently was not going to get this respect from his own father, the time Aaron spent tormenting his father became a game he enjoyed and looked forward to. He enjoyed making his father feel uncomfortable. He no longer felt inferior to or humiliated by his father but felt enough continued anger to torment him. His father hadn't changed, and this game was a continued reminder of Aaron's own new perception of life and a way to remain on guard. The King within prepared him to continue on the path of prudence and humility, to be on guard for old and new monsters in his life.

I saw Peggy about two weeks later. She reported she was no longer waking in the morning tense and exhausted. An obvious change was her new-found ability to nurture others, providing them with "loving support." This change was reflected inwardly with her ability to nurture herself. She faced and awoke the nurturing Queen within her.

To proclaim her victory to the King, she had evidence in her stories of nurturing others. The end of her nightmares was further evidence. Peggy's strong sense of self-confidence was the inner King's response of great assurance and celebration, celebrating the victory as complete.

The "external King" was a bit more cautious. I had no doubt that Peggy's "past life" experience offered a powerful experience in the healing process, and I readily accepted the interpretation that she needed loving support. But I remained curious about the possibility that Peggy was denying some significant emptiness in her current life. This emptiness might be the loss of her father when she was one, resulting in an unconscious feeling of abandonment, a preverbal feeling for a one year old. Peggy's mother recovered quickly from the divorce and never talked of Peggy's father after that. Peggy once thought she found a picture of him but never felt comfortable enough to mention the topic to her mother, nor did she considered questioning anyone else about him. She denied the significance of this loss, but even if the past life experience was no more than a metaphoric expression of the loss of her father, there is no reason to question its effectiveness in causing needed change.

BEDDING DOWN FOR THE NIGHT

After a great feast, the shadow of night falls over Heorot and the Danish king and queen retire to their chamber. Beowulf's attendant leads the traveller to his chamber where he falls asleep.

With our task completed, we can finally relax in a comfortable sleep. This metaphor of sleep was literally true for Peggy. She reported she was sleeping soundly, and for the first time that she could remember, she was waking feeling refreshed and alive.

Aaron's new tormenting relationship with his father was a constant reminder of his change and helped keep him from reverting to old habits. One day this game took on a new meaning when Aaron realized he was now not only his father's tormentor but also his teacher. Aaron's father's torment had started Aaron on this journey of change and thus had taught him an important lesson. Now Aaron had something he could teach his father. Aaron realized that an understanding of love was what his father needed most, and that laughter is a necessary part of love. With this resolution the game continued, but now its malicious flavor was gone. At last Aaron was ready to relax, to get a good night's sleep, and in fact for the first time in a long while he woke in the morning feeling truly rested. Aaron felt his change was complete.

Raymond, too, found peace and understanding facing his tormentors. Though he was living at a distance from his parents, he was now able to enjoy them more fully. He was able to make up for lost time by really appreciating his father's gentle and patient nature. His resentment for his mother likewise diminished. He understood why she did what she did, and appreciated her good qualities. After their talk, Raymond's mother appreciated her husband's gentle and patient nature even more. She had never really put her feelings into words, but his gentle and patient nature was a large part of why she loved him. Raymond slept well.

Sally also found peace and understanding after facing her tormentors. She now felt comfortable in front of Bart. She was able to dress and undress in front of him and even enjoyed his glances, knowing how he loved her. Their sexual life together became much more relaxed and comfortable, rather than the roller coaster ride it had been. Sally was able to sleep comfortably beside the man she could trust.

BEOWULF'S PREPARATION FOR RETURNING HOME

A black raven, the blithe-hearted, cheerfully announces the break of day. Beowulf and his men eagerly busy themselves in preparation for returning home. The hero returns the great sword to Unferth. Though the sword was ineffective in severing the head of the she-beast, he proclaims its excellence, speaking no disparagement of it. When the men are prepared to leave, the prince approaches the throne to announce his intent to return home during this time of peace. Beowulf assures the king that he will always be available if other menaces come into his life.

The purpose of the warrior within is to protect and defend us. With victory, there is no other immediate challenge, so the warrior within prepares to return to his rightful vantage point to be on call for the king. It is important to let down our active defenses so we can live in peace and contentment.

Raymond was about to continue on his journey of life without my weekly support. We decided upon one last session in a month for review. Rather than "trying" to be gentle and patient, he now really felt gentle and patient. I asked Raymond to find something to carry with him to be a constant reminder of his new self. The next week he stopped by with a smooth stone from a nearby river bed, polished by the gentle and patient flow of the water: a gift from the King. He planned to drill a hole in the stone and put it on his keychain.

Aaron, too, was packing up, getting ready to move on. There was something he needed though. His ability to love and respect other men was very much in its infant stage and one sided. He appreciated other men when they expressed appreciation or respect for him, when Bill told him that if anyone could loosen up his father it would be Aaron. But, Aaron had not matured to the point of being able to express appreciation or respect for other men.

Since the end of therapy was rapidly approaching I needed to find a way to insure the gains made so far. This need was filled in a surprising way. Aaron brought to therapy a couple of family pictures including his father, "before" and "after," one with the look of scorn, and a very recent family portrait with his father smiling, a strange forced smile. Aaron took some responsibility for this change even though at times other than a family photograph his father would not be caught smiling. These pictures were an important reminder for Aaron of the influence he had on his father, of his ability to loosen up his father with smiles and laughter.

Sally was ready to end therapy to enjoy her newfound healthy relationship with Bart. She no longer felt crazy and no longer made Bart crazy with her violent mood swings. Her healthy love and sex life with Bart was the gift from the King.

Craig too was ready to end therapy. He came to this last session with a dream. It was a flying dream, a dream of flying under his own power, a dream I find very encouraging. In the dream Craig was flying along the coast of an ocean. "It was a beautiful warm and clear day. I could see for miles. After flying for some time I saw a pier jutting out into the water. A car was driving out onto the pier. I could see there were four people in the car. I decided to land on the pier but it was wet, and as I landed, I slid off and into the water. I came out coughing and spitting water. I climbed up a ladder on the side up the pier. When I got up the four people were getting out of the car. My mother, brother, father, and grandfather. My mother said to my brother, "Why can't you fly like Craig?" My father said, "You shouldn't be flying, you don't have a license." My grandfather said, "Cut out the bellyaching, that was only water." I looked at them with disgust, gave them 'the finger' and flew on," laughing to myself. Craig was prepared to return home.

THE GIFTS FROM THE KING

King Hrothgar praises Beowulf for his strength, wisdom, discretion and impeccability. He vows eternal friendship and the future exchange of gifts in love. At last the King gives Beowulf twelve treasures of the hall and bids him go in peace but return soon.

Why 12 treasures? Twelve represents the complete circle, the number of the moons of the year. "The number twelve, divisiblest of all, which could be halved, quartered, parted into three, into six, the most remarkable number—this was enough to determine the signs of the Zodiac, the number of Odin's sons, and innumerable other twelves," suggests Thomas Carlyle (1908).

These 12 treasures were the "divisiblest of all," thus the king gives Beowulf the whole. We treasure and value our warrior self just this dearly. Our warrior self is our salvation.

Craig had received his 12 treasures. He had overcome the suffering caused by the three tormentors in his life and could now fly under his own power, completing the circle of victory. He could be comfortable in his work and life without the obsessive worry of upsetting or offending others. He was now better equipped for other battles to be fought and victories to be won in the future. He was on his way home.

Megan worked and practiced. We extended the time between therapy sessions first to every two weeks, then to once a month. We talked about her experiences of success and times of back-sliding. Each session included a review of and pep talk about her need to learn to nurture and care for her husband. Megan saw the more she gave to him, the more he gave in return.

About two months later Megan came to a therapy session with an experience. She had gone to the National Gallery of Art and had seen John Singer Sargent's *El Jaleo,* "the uproar." She very much identified with the Spanish dancer who stood among a number of sleepy Spanish musicians and began to dance, stirring to life other dancers at the far right edge of the panting. She very much felt the "uproar" in her life, bringing her femininity alive among a bunch of sleepy men musicians. Her nurturing side became alive. The images of a painting reflected beautifully the completeness of her feelings better than words. This image, *El Jaleo,* became the 12 treasures of the King.

Raymond's gifts were first his new found ability to communicate intimately with his wife. His marriage flourished. Second, he had grown as a manager at work. When he looked back in time he now understood the meaning of being promoted to one's level of incompetency, but he now feels competent as a plant manager, and the ceiling has been removed.

Peggy's obvious gift was her peace of mind while sleeping. Another gift was the power she found from her unconscious mind. Her experience of a past life opened a whole new world to her as a spiritual person. Though I suggested that her experience of a past life does not necessarily prove the existence of a past life, it does prove that the images that can come from the unconscious mind are very important and powerful. Though Peggy did not attribute this experience to God, she took this importance and power of the unconscious mind as something from beyond the ordinary, a spiritual experience that gave her new powers of control over her life.

SETTING SAIL

Beowulf and his men begin the trek to the coast and their waiting vessel. The coastguard meets them with honor as they embark with their bright armor, horses, arms and gold. Beowulf presents a sword to the officer who has guarded the vessel. The ship then sets out to return home.

Now is the time to return to our normal life with a new attitude of self-confidence and contentment. It is time to appreciate and honor the fact this life continues for us. Because of our victory we can appreciate and honor it more than ever. Now is the time to end therapy, at least for the time being.

With the image of *El Jaleo,* Megan ended therapy. She returned home feeling like a new person. Her nurturing and caring side that had seemed dead was now alive, in a glorious uproar, waking the rest of her.

Raymond was on his way. The CEO of his company took notice of him and praised him in handling the downsizing. He suggested that Raymond was in line for a promotion to the larger facility back in the city. This family can now look forward to being back near both sets of parents.

I saw Aaron for one last session about a month later. He continued to feel like a different person. His life was still intact. His relationship with his wife seemed better than ever. He even enjoyed being around his parents. He felt concerned for his father and felt strong in demonstrating to him how life could be different. The barrier to his ability to love men was crumbling, as evident in his insight that he was becoming his father's teacher. Aaron himself had never wanted children, even though his wife did. Now he announced they had decided to start a family. Though his old life was still available to him, in his new life he found not only more contentment and comfort, but also more self-confidence and self-respect.

This next session with Peggy ended with the decision it would be her last. Her life was continuing with Russ and with her work as a paralegal. She was relating well to Russ, nurturing him and receiving nurturance from him. She also nurtured her clients when they needed it. She felt good about her independence from her mother, which in turn allowed their relationship grow and improve. She was sleeping well, no longer bothered by her night terrors. I again offered Peggy the caution, "If something else develops that might trouble you, I will continue to be available." But, in a self-confident manner, she brushed off my offer with a shrug. This time the shrug had a different message. Her new spiritual growth led her to record her dreams and to continue searching her unconscious mind. She knew she would be back to see me with such dreams and other insights.

IN CONCLUSION

Beowulf returns home with great fame as a warrior. Some time later his king, Hygelac, is killed in battle and Beowulf becomes king. Beowulf is a great and benevolent king for fifty years until the day he dies in battle at the claws of a great dragon.

To this point our story has been of Beowulf as the warrior. Yet this story continues with Beowulf as the king. Each of us has a life beyond the battles with Grendel and his mother. Our victory in these battles makes us much stronger and wiser. With continued growth, our wise inner king will attain the strength of Beowulf. We will likely face further torment in our lives but we now can face it with this new strength and wisdom. Most of the six clients of this book did return for a limited number of sessions of therapy for assistance when further torment entered their lives. Continued work can be expected before our inner king becomes established on the firmest ground.

What can we expect in life after our victory? We have learned to face torment with intent, patience, curiosity and gentleness. We can expect life to be more carefree and more loving. We will find greater harmony, tranquility, and satisfaction in life. We will feel stronger and know we have the strength to face and conquer other torments that may come our way.

Will the day come when all torment is conquered? I enjoy contemplating this possibility. What then might life be like? In psychology we talk about the self-actualized person and use such language as "going beyond the ego," and "transpersonal psychology." This language suggests a state of consciousness beyond our usual states of consciousness of which most of us are familiar. Various forms of meditation are taught with the aim of bringing us to this state. This ultimate state has been called by many names: Nirvana, enlightenment, the immortal realm, cosmic consciousness, or heaven. Some writings suggest that in this state beyond we will have powers that would be hard for most of us to even imagine now. Whether we attain this state before or after our life as we know it ends, most religions believe that we can look forward to going beyond with a sense of hope and excitement. We can expect to enjoy life more totally.

Are there other ways to attain this ultimate state? Many writers suggest that this state can be attained simply through some form of meditation or prayer. I tend to believe as Jack Kornfield (1993) does, that even the best meditators have old wounds to heal, and the best avenue to heal these wounds is through a combination of meditation or prayer and psychotherapy. Personal and family history are the sources of these wounds. These wounds simply cannot be ignored and transcended through meditation but need to be uncovered, faced, and healed.

King Beowulf eventually died. During his 50 years as king he gained great wealth, power, and prestige. He left a great legacy for those who followed him.

The six clients of this book have continued to grow. They have continued in their process of uncovering, facing and healing to find greater satisfaction and fulfillment in their lives. Each has learned greater intimacy in their primary relationships with others and these relationships have flourished. These six individuals will not be forgotten in their eventual death. We all must die, but these individuals will be greater inspirations to others in their death than they would have been without having faced their Grendel and His Mother.

References

Araoz, Daniel L. *The New Hypnosis*. New York: Brunner/Mazel, 1985.
Barnett, E. A. *Analytical Hypnotherapy: Principles and Practice*. Kingston, Ontario, Canada: Junica, 1981.
Brink, N. E. The Power Struggle of Workers' Compensation and Strategies for Intervention. *Journal of Applied Rehabilitation Counseling, 20*(1),1989.
Brink, N. E. God Images. In R. G. Kunzendorf (Ed.). *Mental Imagery*. New York: Plenum, 1991.
Brink, N. E. Loki's Children: A Mythical Understanding of Hypnosis in the Process of Change. *Hypnos, 22*(3), 1995.
Buchholz, D. Sleep Disorders. *Treatment Trends: A Newsletter of Taylor Manor Hospital, 3*(1), 1988.
Cantor, Dorothy W., & T. Bernay. *Women in Power: The Secrets of Leadership*. Boston: Houghton Mifflin Co., 1992.
Carlyle, Thomas. *Heroes and Hero Worship: The Heroic in History*. New York: E. P. Dutton, 1908.
Castaneda, Carlos. *Tales of Power*. New York: Pocket Books, 1974.
Dubovsky, Steven L. *Mind Body Deceptions: The Psychosomatics of Everyday Life*. New York: W. W. Norton, 1997.
Erickson, Milton H., E. L. Rossi, & S. I. Rossi. *Hypnotic Realities: The Induction of Clinical Hypnosis and Forms of Indirect Suggestion*. New York: Irvington, 1976.
Kornfield, Jack. Even the Best Meditators Have Old Wounds to Heal: Combining Meditation and Psychotherapy. In R. Walsh & F. Vaughan (Eds.). *Paths Beyond Ego: The Transpersonal Vision* (pp. 67-69). Los Angeles: Jeremy P. Tarcher/Perigee, 1993.
Masterson, James F. *The Search for the Real Self: Unmasking the Personality Disorders of Our Age*. New York: The Free Press, 1988.
Miller, Alice. *The Drama of the Gifted Child: The Search for the True Self*. New York: Basic Books, 1981.
Moore, Robert, & D. Gilette. *King Warrior Magician Lover: Rediscovering the Archetypes of the Mature Masculine*. San Francisco: Harper San Francisco, 1991.
Perls, Frederick S. *Gestalt Therapy Verbatim*. New York: Bantam Books, 1970.
Tavris, Carol. *Anger: The Misunderstood Emotion*. New York: Simon and Schuster, 1982.
Sgroi, Suzanne M. *Vulnerable Populations Volume 2: Sexual Abuse Treatment for Children, Adult Survivors, Offenders, and Persons with Mental Retardation*. Lexington, Mass: Lexington Books, 1989.
Watkins, John G. The Affect Bridge: A Hypnoanalytic Technique, *International Journal of Clinical and Experimental Hypnosis, 19*, pp. 21-27, 1971.

Index

Aaroz, Daniel, 123
Abandonment, 7-22, 23
Abstract Reasoning, lack of, 16
Abuse, 3, 12
Adult-self, 3, 47, 54-55, 73, 78, 97, 101,
    103, 107-108, 110, 114-115, 122,
    140, 141, 150-151, 152-154,
    155-159, 161
Affect bridge, 2-3, **53**-55, 72-73, 77-78,
    114, 129, 139-143, 146, 149, 150,
    151-158
Analytic hypnotherapy, 53-55
Anger, 155
Anxiety, accepting, 66, 119
  cause of, 1, 7, 11, 23, 24, 47, 53, 61, 94,
    105, 114, 146, 153
  facing, 47, 94, 141
  joining, 59, 111
  letting go, 41
  overcoming, 44, 94, 125
  reframing, 42, 98
  seeking safe place, 61
  as unconscious message, 42, 94
Archetypes, 93
Assignments, 125, 160
Autonomic nervous system, 80

Back sliding, 109
Barnett, Edgar, 53, 54
Biofeedback, 43, 45
Bind, 11
Blame, 25-26, 63
Bloom, Peter, 46
Body's defense, 41
Bowlby, John, 13
Breathing, 50

Brink, Nicholas, 28, 31
Buckholtz, D., 45
Burden, carrying a, 95

Cain and Abel, 23-25
Cantor, Dorothy, 15
"Checker," 41
Control, gaining, 17-20
  letting go of, 45, 47-48, 49
Country path, 56-57
Cry for help, 40
Curiosity, 144-145
Curiosity and wonder suggestion, 43, 46,
    50, 53-54, 58, 71-72, 75-76, 77, 78,
    82, 89-90, 99, 114, 151

Defenses, development of, 5-6, 11-20
  letting go of, 5, 33, 45-49, 66, 79-83,
    84-87, 95, 127-128, 130, 140, 176
  natural, 41, 79
  resistance to letting go, 61, 63
Delusion, grandiose, 17
Denial, 45
Dependency, 7
Depression, 5, 7, 22, 42, 46, 55, 59, 68, 72,
    97, 107, 110, 122, 127, 130, 132-133,
    136, 143, 163, 172
Developmental stages, 7-8
Dissociation, 7-8, 15-17, 22, 71-72, 130,
    145, 151
Double bind, 85
Double chair technique, 123, 146
Doors along hallway technique, 56-58
Dreams, meaning of, 1
  remembering, 44-45

Dreamwork, 1-2, 39, 48, 51-52, 60, 65, 74-75, 80, 96, 102-104, 107, 108-109, 111, 120-121, 143, 155

Ego strengthening, 87-88, 105-106, 120, 127-128, 129
Elevator technique, 46, 127-128, 138-139
Emergency response, 80
Emotional incest, 156
Emotional release, 142
Emptiness, facing, 46-47, 85-86, 143-144, 149-150
Empty box, 86-87
Envy, 25-27
Erickson, Milton, 61, 84
Etiquette, 14
Exhibitionist, 65, 67
Extramarital affair, 12, 19, 42, 48, 59-61, 63-64, 67-68, 87-88, 104, 105, 125, 137

Facing tormentor, 79, 97-99, 137-139
"Fake it 'til you make it," 93
False Confidence, 58, 106
False Security, 58, 106
Father archetype, 89, 160-162, 163
Feeling identification, 3, 158-160, 168
Female archetype, 66-69, 126-127, 169
Finger signaling, 3, 54-55, 78, 99, 142, 146
Focusing, 88

Galvanic skin response (GSR), 43
Gentleness, 144-145
Gestalt dreamwork, 2, 4
Giving-up, 33
Gillette, Douglas, 126
God, 10, 11, 23, 24-25, 28-29, 34-35, 52, 75
Grief, 30, 133-135
Guided imagery, 2, 4
Guilt, 60, 65, 78, 130, 140

Habits, 5
Hand levitation, 76

History taking, 51
Hypnotic assignments, 125
Hypnotic monologue, 47, 58, 64, 65, 69, 96-97, 125, 134, 135, 136, 137, 138, 145, 163-164, 171, 172
Hypnotic rehearsal, 55, 56, 74, 83, 87-88, 115
Hypnotic strategies, 1-2

Identifying feelings, 3, 158-160, 168
Identifying needs, 3, 140-141, 160-162, 168
Imagery, 86-87, 104-105, 111, 119, 146, 150
Imposter, 30
Incest, 158-159
Inner mother, 66-69, 126-127, 142, 160, 162
Inner father, 89, 141-142, 160-162
Insight, 75-76
Intent, 144-145
Intuition, 130

Joining, 59, 63, 129, 133-134
Journaling, 142, 160-161, 162
Jung, Karl, 4

King archetype, 71, 121, 126

Letting go, 40, 47-48, 76-77
Loneliness, 9-10
Love, conditional/unconditional, 48, 64, 73, 76, 86-87, 137

Magical thinking, 35-36
Male archetype, 66-67, 126-127
Marital discord, 5
Masterson, James, 13
Memorializing, 116
Miller, Alice, 9, 22
Moore, Robert, 126
Mother archetype, 163

Mountain path technique, 117-118
Myth, 4
Myth, global understanding, 4

Nagual, 75
Narcissist, 13
Need identification, 140-141, 160-162, 168
Nightmares, 44-45, 149
Night terrors, 44, 49, 53, 89, 94
"No" response, 47
Nothingness, facing, 46-47, 85-86, 143-144, 149-150
Nurturance, 66-69

Obsessions, 6, 7, 41
Obsessive-compulsive, 32-33, 41-42
Obsessive worry, 30, 34-35, 56, 77, 89, 93-94, 105, 113-115, 130, 134, 161, 162

Pain, 31-32, 95, 100-102, 103, 149, 152
Parasympathetic nervous system, 80
Passive, 7
Past life regression, 156, 158, 164-167, 171
Pacing, 64
Panic, 29, 31, 32, 44, 49, 50, 53, 61, 77, 80, 98, 103-105, 132, 149
Perfectionist, 11-12
Perls, Fritz, 2
Phobias, 7
Physical abuse, 8, 10
Power struggle, 32, 84-85
Psyching up, 56, 88

Rapport, 40-45, 59
Reassurance, 40, 44, 59
Redreaming, 96
Reframing, 41-43, 49-50, 76, 86, 88, 104
Regression, 2-3, 53-55, 72-73, 77, 78, 94, 99-101, 106, 110-111, 114, 129, 139-143, 146, 149, 151-158
Rehearsal, 55, 56, 74, 83, 87-88, 115

Relaxation exercise, 2, 49-50, 53-54, 67, 80, 83, 89-90, 100, 136
Resistance, 47, 63-64, 129, 142, 153
Responsibility, 43, 54, 56, 72-73, 80-82, 94-95, 96, 100-102, 109, 111, 134
Rossi, Ernest, 61

Safe place, 61-62
Sargent, Norah, 28
Saving face, 59, 60-61
Schizophrenia, 17
Secondary gain, 85, 94
Seeing nothing, 46-47, 85-86, 143-144, 149-150
Seeking to please, 13-15
Seduction, 65-66, 67, 74
Self-blame, 27-28
Sexual abuse, 8, 10, 155-156, 169
Shoulder pain, 95, 100-102, 103, 152
Smoking habit, 84-85, 88, 129
Suicide, 33-34, 59
Symbols of change, 113, 116, 120, 121, 125, 126, 176-178
Sympathetic nervous system, 80, 84

Tavris, Carol, 14
Temper tantrum, 7
Time regression, 2-3, 53-55, 72-73, 77, 78, 94, 99-101, 106, 110-111, 114, 129, 139-143, 146, 149, 151-158
Tonal, 75
Tormentor, 5, 29, 45
  facing, 42, 56-58, 76, 84, 89-90, 98, 107, 135, 145, 155, 158, 162, 167, 175
Trance induction, 46, 49-50, 53-54, 83-85, 89, 94, 100
Trauma, 1, 4-5, 7-22, 80
  nature of, 8-10
  survival from, 10
Trust, 40, 42, 43, 45, 49, 79
  lack of, 73
Type-A personality, 11-12, 18
Tyrant king, 73

Unconscious, accessing, 1, 3, 39, 40, 41, 94
  beliefs, 106
  fear of, 71
  gifts, 178
  mind, 1, 22, 34-35, 39-41, 53, 77, 79, 94, 107, 119, 141, 178
  journey into, 138-139, 141-142, 145-146, 149-155, 179
  making, 119-121, 124-126
  messages, 1, 23-24, 39-42, 50, 53, 76, 79, 90, 94, 129, 136, 138, 172-174
  processes, 2, 3, 4
  self-image, 1
Uncovery, 6, 12, 27, 29, 61, 63, 76, 118, 129, 133, 135, 140, 142, 145, 158
Unknown, venturing into, 71-72, 74, 75, 79, 149, 152

Validation, 45, 49

Walking down steps technique, 53-54
Wall, 57, 77
Warrior archetype, 72, 126, 176
Warrior within, 40-41, 42, 45, 136
Watkins, John, 53
Willpower, 1, 45, 48, 50, 95, 106 123
Withdrawal, 32

Yes-set, 61, 64, 69, 84, 134
Younger-self, 3, 47, 54-55, 73, 78, 89 97, 107-108, 110, 114-115, 122, 140, 141, 150- 151, 152-154, 155-159

Other Titles in the
Imagery and Human Development Series
Series Editor, Anees A. Sheikh

Handbook of Therapeutic Imagery Techniques
edited by Anees A. Sheikh

Healing Images: The Role of Imagination in Health
edited by Anees A. Sheikh

The Psychophysiology of Mental Imagery: Theory, Research and Application
edited by Robert G. Kunzendorf and Anees A. Sheikh

Individual Differences in Imaging: Their Measurement, Origins, and Consequences
Alan Richardson

Dream Images: A Call to Mental Arms
edited by Jayne Gackenbach and Anees A. Sheikh

Imagery in Sports and Physical Performance
edited by Anees A. Sheikh and Errol R. Korn

Hypnosis and Imagination
edited by Robert G. Kunzendorf, Nicholas P. Spanos, and Benjamin Wallace

For Product Safety Concerns and Information please contact our EU
representative GPSR@taylorandfrancis.com
Taylor & Francis Verlag GmbH, Kaufingerstraße 24, 80331 München, Germany

www.ingramcontent.com/pod-product-compliance
Lightning Source LLC
Chambersburg PA
CBHW050635300426
44112CB00012B/1803